DATA-DRIVEN ANALYTICS FOR HEALTHCARE

Artificial Intelligence and Machine Learning for Medical Diagnostics

DATA-DRIVEN ANALYTICS FOR HEALTHCARE

Artificial Intelligence and Machine Learning for Medical Diagnostics

Meghna Sharma, PhD
Priyanka Vashisht, PhD
A. V. Senthil Kumar, PhD
Chitra Singh, PhD
Abdelmalek Amine, PhD
Editors

AAP APPLE ACADEMIC PRESS

First edition published 2025

Apple Academic Press Inc.
1265 Goldenrod Circle, NE,
Palm Bay, FL 32905 USA

760 Laurentian Drive, Unit 19,
Burlington, ON L7N 0A4, CANADA

CRC Press
2385 NW Executive Center Drive,
Suite 320, Boca Raton FL 33431

4 Park Square, Milton Park,
Abingdon, Oxon, OX14 4RN UK

Library and Archives Canada Cataloguing in Publication

CIP data on file with Canada Library and Archives

Library of Congress Cataloging-in-Publication Data

CIP data on file with US Library of Congress

ISBN: 978-1-77491-760-2 (hbk)
ISBN: 978-1-77491-761-9 (pbk)
ISBN: 978-1-00355-874-3 (ebk)

About the Editors

Meghna Sharma, PhD
Associate Professor and Data Science Specialisation Lead,
Department of Computer Science and Engineering,
The NorthCap University, Gurugram, Haryana, India

Meghna Sharma, PhD, is currently working as an Associate Professor and Data Science Specialisation Lead in the Department of Computer Science and Engineering at The NorthCap University (NCU), Gurugram, India. She has more than 20 years of teaching, research, and administration experience. Dr. Sharma has worked as a Scientist in the Control Systems Group, ISRO Satellite Center, Bangalore. She is a recipient of 'Award for Science' conferred by Govt. of Haryana. Her major areas of interests are machine learning, artificial intelligence, big data analytics, and data mining. She has more than 35 research papers to her credit published in reputed journals, conferences, and book chapters. She has three international patents published and granted and two national patents published in the AI domain. She has also been a participant in the program committees of several international conferences and on the editorial boards of eminent international journals. She has many certification courses of cutting-edge technologies in the domain of data science to her credit from international and national universities of repute through NPTEL, Coursera, and UpGrad. She has obtained her Doctor of Philosophy in the area of Machine Learning from J.C. Bose University of Science and Technology, YMCA, India.

Priyanka Vashisht, PhD
Associate Professor, Department of Computer Science and Engineering,
Amity University Haryana, Gurugram, India

Priyanka Vashisht, PhD, is currently working as an Associate Professor in the Department of Computer Science & Engineering at Amity University Haryana, Gurugram, India. Her major areas of interests are cloud computing, fog computing, machine learning, big data analytics, and data mining. She has more than 19 years of teaching, research, and administration experience. She is a member of the Association for Computing Machinery (ACM) and faculty sponsor for the ACM Students Chapter. She has numerous research papers to her credit published in reputed journals, conferences, as well as book chapters. She has two Indian and two international patents in her name. She is associated with several computer science journals. She has chaired various international conferences and is a reviewer for many national and international conferences and journals. She earned her doctorate degree in Grid Computing from Thapar University, Patiala, India, in 2017.

A. V. Senthil Kumar, PhD
Director and Professor, Department of Research and PG in Computer Applications, Hindusthan College of Arts and Science, Coimbatore, Tamil Nadu, India

A. V. Senthil Kumar, PhD, is currently designated as Director and Professor in the Department of Research and PG in Computer Applications, Hindustan College of Arts and Science, Tamil Nadu, India. He has industrial experience of five years and teaching experience of 27 years. He has to his credit 33 book chapters, 220 papers in international and national journals, 60 papers in international and national conferences, and edited 12 books (IGI Global, USA). He is an Associate Editor of *IEEE Access*. He is an editor-in-chief for many journals and a key member for the Machine Intelligence Research Lab (MIR Labs), India. Professor Kumar is an editorial board member and reviewer for various international journals. He is also a committee member for various international conferences. He is a life member of the International Association of Engineers (IAENG) and Systems Society of India (SSI) and a member of the Indian Science Congress Association, Internet Society (ISOC), International Association of Computer Science and Information Technology (IACSIT), Indian Association for Research in Computing Science (IARCS), and committee member for various international conferences. He has received his Doctor of Science (DSc in Computer Science).

Chitra Singh, PhD
Professor, Department of Chemistry Education and Environmental Education, National Council of Educational Research and Training (NCERT), Bhopal, Madhya Pradesh, India

Chitra Singh, PhD, has been working as a Professor in the Department of Chemistry Education and Environmental Education at the National Council of Educational Research and Training (NCERT) in Bhopal, Madhya Pradesh, India, for more than 22 years. Dr. Singh has published more than 40 papers in journals, completed eight research projects, conducted 25 training programs, and developed 20 curriculum materials.

Abdelmalek Amine, PhD
Full Professor in Computer Science, Director of Knowledge Management and Complex Data Laboratory (GeCoDe Lab), and Vice Rector of External Relations and Cooperation, Dr. Moulay Tahar Université de Saida, Algeria

Abdelmalek Amine, PhD, is a full Professor of Computer Science at the University of Saida Dr. Moulay Tahar, Algeria, where he is also Director of the Knowledge Management and Complex Data Laboratory (GeCoDe Lab) andVice Rector of External Relations and Cooperation. His research interests include big data, IoT, data mining, text mining, ontology, classification, clustering, neural networks, and biomimetic optimization methods. He has several publications (articles, chapters, and edited books) in the field of AI. He has also been a participant in the program committees of several international conferences and is on the editorial boards of eminent international journals.

Contents

Contributors

A. Aishwariya
Research Scholar, Department of Electronics and Instrumentation Engineering, SRM Institute of Science and Technology, Chennai, Tamil Nadu, India

Gurjapna Anand
Department of Computer Science and Engineering, Amity University, Gurgaon, Haryana, India

Balaganesh
Professor, Computer Science and Multimedia, Lincoln University College, Malaysia

A. B. Bhattacharya
Brainware University, Barasat, Kolkata, West Bengal, India

Arkajit Bhattacharya
Indian Institute of Engineering Science and Technology, Institute Hospital Unit, Shibpur, Howrah, West Bengal, India

Mani Butwall
Assistant Professor, Department of CSE, SKIT, Jaipur, Rajasthan, India

H. R. Chennamma
JSS Science and Technology University, Mysore, Karnataka, India

Uma N. Dulhare
Muffakham Jah College of Engineering and Technology, Hyderabad, Telangana, India

Jai Gaur
Department of IT, Bhagwan Parshuram Institute of Technology, Delhi, India

Shailendra Singh Gaur
Department of IT, Bhagwan Parshuram Institute of Technology, Delhi, India

Sarthak Goel
School of Information Technology and Engineering, Vellore Institute of Technology, Vellore, Tamil Nadu, India

Anamika Guha
School of Information Technology and Engineering, Vellore Institute of Technology, Vellore, Tamil Nadu, India

Vansh Gupta
Department of IT, Bhagwan Parshuram Institute of Technology, Delhi, India

Mohammed Ali Hussain
Professor and Associate Dean R&D, KLEF (Deemed to be University), Guntur, Andhra Pradesh, India

A. V. Senthil Kumar
Professor, Department of MCA, Hindusthan College of Arts and Science, Coimbatore, Tamil Nadu, India

R. Bagavathi Lakshmi
Assistant Professor, Department of Computer Applications, Mannar Thirumalai Naicker College, Tamil Nadu, India

B. Madhushree
JSS Science and Technology University, Mysore, Karnataka, India

K. T. Magesh
Vice Principal and Head, Department of Oral Pathology and Microbiology, SRM Kattankulathur Dental College and Hospital, Tamil Nadu, India

B. Malavika
Department of MCA, Hindusthan College of Arts and Science, Coimbatore, Tamil Nadu, India

Shaik Khaja Mohiddin
Postdoctoral Fellow, Lincoln University College, Malaysia

Shaik Rasool
Methodist College of Engineering and Technology, Hyderabad, Telangana, India

A. Saranya
Guest Lecturer, Department of Computer Applications, Madurai Kamaraj University, Tamil Nadu, India

Ruchi Sehrawat
Department of Computer Science, University School of Information, Communication, and Technology, Guru Gobind Singh Indraprastha University, Delhi, India

Meenakshi Sharma
Assistant Professor-SS, University of Petroleum and Energy Studies, Dehradun, Uttarakhand, India

Priyanka Sharma
Assistant Professor, Department of CSE, SKIT, Jaipur, Rajasthan, India

K. A. Sunitha
Associate Professor and Head, Department of Electronics and Communication Engineering, SRM University, Andhra Pradesh, India

B. K. Tripathy
School of Information Technology and Engineering, Vellore Institute of Technology, Vellore, Tamil Nadu, India

G. Vanishree
Faculty, IBS, Bangalore, Karnataka, India

Tanishq Varshney
Department of Computer Science, University School of Information, Communication, and Technology, Guru Gobind Singh Indraprastha University, Delhi, India

Priyanka Vashisht
Associate Professor, Department of Computer Science and Engineering, Amity University Haryana, Gurugram, India

Preface

The book aims to provide insight into various solutions to diagnose patients with the help of an automated process using artificial intelligence techniques and technology. The emergence of advanced analytics, machine learning, and artificial intelligence techniques provides various possibilities for transforming this data into a form that can help in the process of decision-making, provide high-quality patient care, respond to real-time situations, and save more lives in the clinical front. It will also optimize the use of resources, improve the processes and services, and reduce the costs on the operational and financial front. Intelligent systems cannot replace doctors or human clinicians completely but surely can assist them in diagnosing and giving prognoses with good accuracy and at a large scale. The changing trends are quite evident, considering the current scenario in the healthcare domain where numerous automated tools based on artificial intelligence are used for faster diagnosis and treatment.

Data-driven analytics in healthcare can automate the prediction process so that it can help doctors formulate more effective treatment plans. This book targets those who are pursuing research in healthcare, stakeholders of the healthcare industry, as well as the users of the technology. Data-driven medicine unlocks the avenues of personalized medical treatments with great speed and accuracy. This book highlights the possibilities of artificial intelligence, machine learning, and deep learning techniques, and various tools to correctly diagnose various medical problems, thus easing the burden of doctors and medical staff. It explores the opportunities in data-driven analytics for healthcare in terms of research conducted in this domain and how the data in various healthcare-related applications can be handled and used.

There are general predictive analysis methods explained in various disease detection applications along with machine learning techniques for the implementation of predictive analysis methods. How the human brain can be used as a quantum computer for biomimetics and the mind-machine interface are explained here. One chapter describes various object detection approaches for diseases such as pneumonia, a very common side effect of COVID-19. An application for monitoring and tracking corona disease is also discussed in detail. Various endodontic applications handling diagnostic abnormalities using deep learning methods are explained. An application of healthcare for human activity recognition is also discussed in one of the chapters.

This book is written for a broad audience of those interested in the applications of artificial intelligence and machine learning for various medical applications, such as MRI, X-ray, CT scan image diagnosis, as well as to understand and study the effect of various attributes of the patients as recorded in the patients' history data for diseases prediction, prescription of various drugs, correlation among various attributes, etc.

This book helps computer scientists, electronics engineers, and bioinformatics, pharmaceuticals professionals and doctors, researchers, biotech professionals in adopting artificial intelligence, machine learning. The focus is that artificial intelligence will help unlock the power of big data and gain insight into patients, coordinate care and foster communication at low cost, and help the researchers update the various methods of disease detection and prevention techniques in an early stage to save the lives of people.

Introduction

Data-driven healthcare analytics is a multidisciplinary field that combines advanced technology, statistical modeling, and medical expertise to generate insights into healthcare delivery, patient outcomes, and disease trends. This area is rapidly growing, driven by the increasing availability of electronic health records, medical imaging, and other sources of healthcare data.

Data-driven analytics helps healthcare providers and researchers identify patterns and correlations in large datasets that are too complex for human analysis. It involves developing mathematical models and algorithms to process and analyze vast amounts of data, leading to the identification of trends, patterns, and relationships.

One of the significant benefits of data-driven healthcare analytics is improving patient outcomes. Healthcare providers can develop personalized treatment plans by analyzing data from electronic health records, clinical trials, and medical imaging, identifying high-risk patients. This information can also help identify gaps in care, such as missed follow-up appointments or medication noncompliance, which can be addressed to improve patient outcomes.

Another essential application of data-driven healthcare analytics is improving the overall efficiency and effectiveness of healthcare delivery. Healthcare providers can optimize their operations and reduce costs while improving patient satisfaction by analyzing data on patient wait times, resource utilization, and other factors.

Data-driven healthcare analytics also play a vital role in public health by enabling researchers to identify disease trends and risk factors and develop more effective strategies for prevention and treatment.

The global healthcare analytics market was valued at $14.0 billion in 2019 and is expected to reach $50.5 billion by 2026. Healthcare data is projected to grow at a compound annual growth rate of 36% from 2019 to 2025, making it one of the fastest-growing types of data. Machine learning algorithms can predict patient outcomes, such as hospital readmissions and mortality rates, with a high degree of accuracy.

Data-driven healthcare analytics is not only used for clinical decision-making but also for operational and financial decision-making, such as optimizing hospital staffing and reducing healthcare costs. Electronic health records (EHRs) have enabled the collection and analysis of vast amounts of healthcare data, paving the way for data-driven healthcare analytics.

Data-driven healthcare analytics has the potential to transform the healthcare industry, leading to more efficient and effective healthcare delivery, better patient outcomes, and, ultimately, a healthier population. With the help of machine learning and artificial intelligence, healthcare providers can analyze vast amounts of data in real time, making it possible to quickly identify and respond to emerging health threats and improve patient outcomes.

However, data-driven healthcare analytics also presents significant challenges, such as ensuring the privacy and security of patient data. Healthcare providers must take steps to safeguard patient data while ensuring that it is used ethically and transparently.

Overall, data-driven healthcare analytics offers many benefits, but it must be implemented and used with care. The impact of data-driven healthcare analytics can be seen as both a boon and a bane, depending on how it is used. While it can provide numerous benefits to patients and healthcare providers, it also raises concerns about transparency, fairness, and accountability. By considering patient privacy, transparency, and ethical concerns, data-driven healthcare analytics has the potential to revolutionize healthcare delivery and improve patient outcomes.

CHAPTER 1

Predictive and Descriptive Analytics in Healthcare

GURJAPNA ANAND and PRIYANKA VASHISHT

Department of Computer Science and Engineering, Amity University Haryana, Gurugram, India

ABSTRACT

Predictive and descriptive analysis of diseases play a dynamic role, especially in the medical industry where predicting diseases reduces the risk that is likely to happen in patients. In the medical field, determining the suitable disease is crucial from the beginning of the patient's journey until the end of any therapy. In the medical industry, the predictive and descriptive analysis of disease is established as a valuable and productive method for advanced diagnosing and taking appropriate action. Descriptive analysis takes advantage of past data, whereas predictive analysis focuses more on future predictions. Predictive analysis is a critical step to prevent any enduring disease, allowing providers to diagnose early symptoms of the ailment. With the help of predictive analysis, it is better to understand the root cause of the disease well in advance. In this study, various frameworks suggested by scholars have been examined, and comparative analysis has been used to gain a better understanding of real-world medical issues. The role of artificial intelligence in predictive and descriptive analysis can be used as a great factor to minimize the risk of disease. It also focuses on diagnosing the disease, such as how artificial intelligence analysis can be combined to improve the patient's journey. Artificial Intelligence uses data to predict the transfer rate of the ICU, which further helps in determining the patient's risk of being prone to infections.

Data-Driven Analytics for Healthcare: Artificial Intelligence and Machine Learning for Medical Diagnostics.
Meghna Sharma, Priyanka Vashisht, A. V. Senthil Kumar, Chitra Singh, and Abdelmalek Amine (Eds.)

1.1 INTRODUCTION

Technological innovation has fast-tracked the expansion of health systems [1] which have completely digitally evolved, and these services include mobile wellbeing or mobile health, health information technology, wearable handsets, telehealth, and personalized medication. This equipment produces a huge amount of data. To manage such a huge amount of data, we need to identify relevant data from a large volume of data by applying analytics.

Analytics is the procedure of exploring the raw datasets to discover new or latest trends, draw decisions, and identify possible improvements in the field of healthcare [5]. Healthcare analytics customize the existing and ancient data to gather the visions, macro, and micro, and conclude with the result at both the patient and commercial level.

These skills are planned to privilege the users to make up-to-date decisions about the anticipation, early recognition, analysis, action, and supervision of numerous severe and long-lasting health [6] problems. A grave component of these numeracy health resolutions is prediction, which is vital to most decision-making developments. Prediction is usually the method of gathering absent evidence by gauging the past data, the existing statistics at present, and the intended data which is achievable soon. In the healthcare domain, reducing all the complex data will never recover persistent patient care unless actionable visions are identified.

The three prime reasons to gain actionable visions using predictive and descriptive analytics [2] in the healthcare sector are as follows:

- The quality of patient care can be improved by using evidence-based medications to inform clinical decisions.
- By predicting the risks associated with a patient's disease, it reduces major healthcare costs.
- It reduces readmissions, and the number of tests for a patient, and also improves hospital-related processes.

Data Analytics and Artificial Intelligence in healthcare play a vital role in defining the good health of a patient, faster and more accurate analysis, defensive actions, personalized treatment, and more convincing outcomes. In the healthcare sector, there are ample records, research papers, and online and offline courses available that provide comprehensive experience in the implementation of AI and data analytics separately. However, there are not many records available that present the application-oriented behavior of predictive [10] and descriptive analytics in the healthcare [8] sector. Such records would be of great help to the readers to understand where AI and Data analytics can be effectively and simultaneously useful in healthcare.

There are certain concerns which may arise when diagnosing a specific disease, as described below:

- What type of data should be collected—medical, social, personal, population health-related—to predict the risk associated with the disease?
- How should the collected data be stored or arranged – to utilize the outcome of the data more productively?
- How can predictive analysis (PA) and descriptive analysis (DA) be useful in predicting early changes in lifestyle or detecting disease symptoms?
- After diagnosing the disease, through what different ways can these two analysis models help in improving the treatment of the disease?

This chapter aims to deliver wide-ranging information about where and how PA and DA can be of use and also their current applications in diversified healthcare areas so that the person who reads can gain knowledge of the aforementioned concerns in their specific field of awareness. The focus of this chapter will be on reviewing and scrutinizing the existing and forthcoming analytics applications in a few healthcare disciplines.

Section 1.2 of this chapter will describe the role of artificial intelligence in the healthcare domain. Section 1.3 of this chapter will describe the role of data analytics in the healthcare domain. Section 1.4 of this chapter will familiarize you in detail with the types of healthcare analytics. Section 1.5 will explain the predictive analysis framework in detail and Section 1.6 will explain the descriptive analysis framework [24] in detail. Section 1.7 focuses on the conclusion of the entire chapter on how Artificial Intelligence and Data Analytics lead to healthcare resolutions.

1.2 ROLE OF ARTIFICIAL INTELLIGENCE IN HEALTHCARE

Predictive and descriptive analysis can be accomplished using simple and complex methods that can be assessed by humans. However, there have been ample scientific developments ongoing in the domain of artificial intelligence (AI) and medical data mining [3]. AI in the healthcare domain is progressively growing. Nowadays, various machine learning, deep learning, expert systems, and natural language processing (NLP) techniques are explored to predict more defined and exhaustive outcomes using predictive and descriptive models. According to S. Poornima and M. Pushpalatha [26], AI has proved to be of great use in the field of healthcare domain [22] because of the following reasons:

- People are more aware of the new technology-driven healthcare domain compared to the old healthcare model [27].
- There is more demand for network-based smart devices in our day-to-day life.
- There is more availability and need for at-home facilities, such as monitoring health issues remotely and telemedicine.

The advantages of incorporating AI into healthcare are more favorable. A huge amount of time and effort is invested in collecting and storing data from various sources.

- Call logs of the customers;
- Medical documents;
- Surveys conducted for the level of satisfaction attained;
- Data produced related to the patient's data.

The application of effective and efficient analytics to convert such complex data into actionable medical [21] intelligence is of great importance. Measures for securing the data have been defined well in advance using both descriptive and predictive analytics [4]. The disadvantage of both predictive and descriptive methods of analytics is that they do not consider forecasting. AI [29] permits predictive and descriptive analytics to produce faster, smarter, and more actionable outcomes. Now, it can be easily comprehended to what extent artificial intelligence plays a major role in the healthcare sector and further it can illustrate how data analytics can have great significance.

1.3 ROLE OF DATA ANALYTICS IN HEALTHCARE

Collecting and storing the data effectively and efficiently is one of the major tasks in the healthcare field. Data will be of no use until it is collected and stored appropriately. For this, a centralized and systematic way must be adopted to better analyze the data, which can be further utilized for any additional purposes.

In recent years, the process of collecting healthcare [20] data has become more organized and modernized. Well-organized data has proven to be beneficial for day-to-day operations and for improving patient care [11]. By examining both historical data and existing evidence, one can easily utilize both datasets to fill any gaps and make advanced predictions. One major advantage of analyzing the data is that precautionary measures can be considered, making subsequent inferences easier.

There is a growing demand for persistent patient-centric services, value-based services, and easily accessible medical care, leading to a significant shift towards predictive [7] and preventive measures in public health in recent years. With the help of data analytics, physicians can identify patients at high risk of developing chronic diseases and provide assistance before it is too late to treat the disease. Additionally, it also reduces costs for practitioners, insurance companies, and hospitalization expenses.

1.4 TYPES OF HEALTHCARE ANALYTICS

In this chapter, we are stressing two kinds of analytics that play a critical role in the healthcare [19] domain, namely predictive analysis (PA) and descriptive analysis (DA).

Predictive analytics will help assess an organization to have a better understanding of the near future, predicting what might occur next. It uses existing data to forecast the future. By analyzing the data, it can provide new conclusions. Predictions are probabilistic and cover all categories.

Descriptive analytics helps assess an organization to understand what has happened in previous years. It analyzes past data collected and stored for further assessment and conclusions. It is important for an organization to identify past events to make better decisions based on historical data. For example, collecting a person's complete medical history is crucial to understanding the patient's condition and taking appropriate action.

As mentioned, there are two types of healthcare analytics, and their comparative study has been conducted based on various parameters such as procedures involved, capacity, accuracy, and methods adopted, presented in Table 1.1.

1.5 PREDICTIVE ANALYTICS FRAMEWORK

The predictive analysis framework makes use of past data for optimal analysis. It has three stages as shown in Figure 1.1.

- Strategy;
- Build;
- Implement.

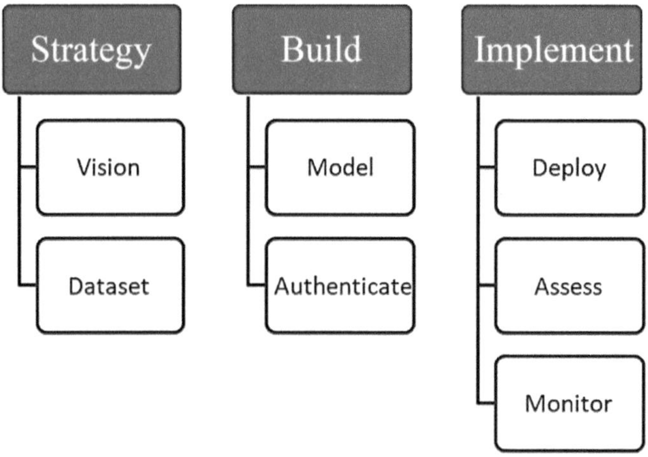

FIGURE 1.1 Stages in predictive analysis framework.

1.5.1 STRATEGY BEHIND THE MODEL

This is the first and one of the most important stages in predictive analysis. In this phase, a vision for the model is decided upon. Also, the procedure to select the datasets for accurate analysis is determined. Various sources need to be considered for the final datasets which are further used for building the model. The detailed work is given in subsections.

1.5.1.1 VISION

A strong, precise vision for the model is essential. Every model is established for its definite reason which cannot be utilized successfully in some other condition. For instance, a model used to forecast online e-commerce clients' churn of the original data (of what PA or DA or something else) cannot be fruitful for predicting credit card-related information. For example, if

TABLE 1.1 . Comparative Study between Predictive Analytics and Descriptive Analytics

Basis for Comparison	Descriptive Analytics	Predictive Analytics
Defines	What occurred in the past? It makes use of the stored data.	What is more likely to happen in the near future? It makes use of the past data and then analyzes it for further use.
Procedure involved	Comprises data aggregation and data mining.	Comprises statistics and forecast methods.
Description	It involves the process of identifying valuable and vital statistics after examining the enormous data.	It involves the process of predicting the future by assessing existing or present data only.
Data capacity	It processes the complex and large data that is kept in the warehouse. It has Limited access to historical data.	It processes complex and large past data and then forecasts the forthcoming by using advanced practices.
Instances	Sales report, company revenue, analyzing performance, etc.	Credit score analysis, Sentimental analysis, company forecast reports, etc. [9]
Correctness	It delivers precise and correct data only.	Conclusions are not that precise and accurate clearly; they will not tell you what will happen, but they will help to make you aware of the events going to happen in the near future.
Method	It follows a reactive and responsive approach.	It follows a proactive and practical approach.

an organization is experiencing a great number of infections, predictive analytics would be of great help here as it will detect which ICU patients could be next on the list according to their vital status, and would also by default identify the specific nurse who could be the root cause for spreading the infection, and proper hygiene and sanitation needs to be followed.

1.5.1.2 PREPARE THE DATASET

The created dataset can roughly cover diversified information like data related to product details, behavioral information, and topographical, geographical, and climatic conditions. The data not considered while preparing the dataset will not be used for making any kind of predictions. All team members, including professional and commercial individuals, participate equally in all sorts of decisions for the dataset creation. The emphasis is more on the behavioral evidence as this is more influential in making any judgments.

1.5.2 BUILD THE MODEL

This phase comprises designing or developing the proposed or filtered model and then validating it for more accuracy and optimization. It generally involves around 20–25% of the total time. It has 2 sub-phases, namely, Model and then Authenticate.

1.5.2.1 MODEL

The designing of the model will be done with the help of the created dataset. There are many factors that are considered, and some of them are not considered while building the model. Few factors are discarded as they might hold little or no information useful for prediction.

1.5.2.2 AUTHENTICATE

Validating the designed or developed model is one of the major and critical phases. As it not only validates against the valid dataset but also against the invalid group of datasets that are not involved in the development of the model.

1.5.3 IMPLEMENT THE MODEL

After planning and building the model, it's finally time to implement and then deploy the designed model. The applicability of the designed model to real-life scenarios can be validated. It serves all business purposes, including the performance of the model, validating, and monitoring the model under certain conditions. This phase is further divided into sub-phases, namely Deploy, Evaluate, and Control. This phase normally takes around 40% of the overall time.

1.5.3.1 DEPLOY THE DESIGNED MODEL

It's time to assess the applicability of the model. It is developed on the basis of a subset of the complete data or dataset. After the data has been validated, it will be used to execute it over the client.

1.5.3.2 ASSESS

In this phase, the performance of the developed model is a major aim to focus on. The predictions will be more accurate if and only if the predictions are done keeping the group of both valid and invalid customers' points of view only.

1.5.3.3 MONITOR

Monitoring the model is a very important phase. It is an ongoing process that never stops at any point in time. How often the model must be monitored, or the duration of monitoring is also considered here. The model must be monitored based on the new data or practices, and methods as they become readily available.

1.6 DESCRIPTIVE ANALYSIS FRAMEWORK

The descriptive analysis framework makes use of the stored data for optimal analysis. It follows a top-to-bottom approach. It is divided into five stages as shown in Figure 1.2.

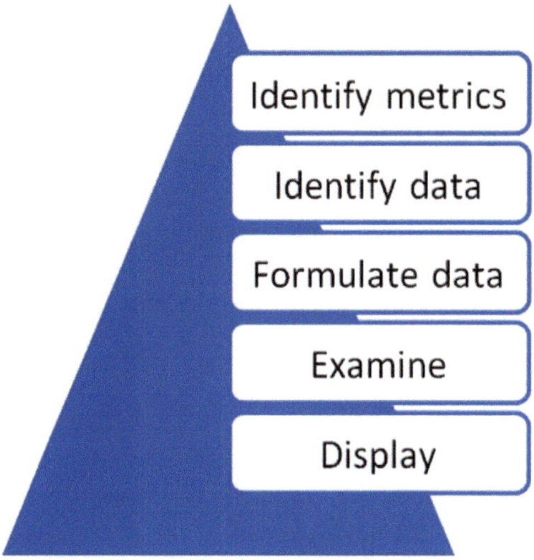

FIGURE 1.2 Stages in descriptive analysis framework.

1.6.1 GAUGE BUSINESS METRICS

The primary step is to recognize the metrics that we wish to populate. All selected metrics must have some primary professional goal. For example, a more development-focused company might emphasize estimating its revenue quarterly instead of daily.

1.6.2 FIND THE REQUIRED DATA

Trace the anticipated data which becomes an output for the chosen metrics. Data must be correctly identified with the appropriate approach [18] as it is always in scattered form. Data might be fetched from some outside agencies or sources like online e-commerce websites, and many social media platforms.

1.6.3 PULLING AND FORMULATING THE DATA

The main aim behind this stage is to ensure that accuracy is achieved anyhow. As data is being collected from many resources obtaining the correct data is a big challenge [24]. So, this entire process is time-consuming. It involves pulling an ample amount of data and then filtering or cleaning the unwanted, irrelevant, inconsistent, and full of error data.

1.6.4 EXAMINE THE DATA

Normally, organizations make use of many analytics tools or software to examine or assess the data. Companies make use of a variety of tools to apply descriptive analytics, from spreadsheets to business intelligence (BI) software.

1.6.5 DISPLAY THE DATA

The most effective way to display the data is in visual forms, such as all types of charts (pie charts, etc.), and graphs. It is the easiest form for the investors, sponsors, and stakeholders to understand the entire populated dataset.

1.7 ADVANTAGES OF AI AND DATA ANALYTICS

The advantages of introducing AI and data analytics into the healthcare area are as mentioned in the subsections:

1.7.1 PREDICTIVE MODELING

The process of examining [23] the present and historical data or information to better predict future outputs. This model makes use of machine learning, data mining, and statistics to recognize the patterns and forecast the results. It offers resolutions on the macro- and micro-levels only.

By using AI and data analytics, healthcare [27] specialists can be mindful of their potential to adapt to risk. The process includes analyzing the communicative data, which will be useful to predict the outcome of the treatment, and probable danger pertaining to enduring illness. The collected health-related data can be used to keep count of the risk, predict the number of readmissions and deterrence, expect infection and deterioration rate, etc.

Predictive modeling is generally used on a much bigger scale. Managing all health-related concerns is impossible without considering this model. Outbursts can be predicted, occurrences can be predicted, results can be predicted, and based on these predictions accordingly preventive measures can be considered. Predictive modeling can even be used in many other kinds of applications to upsurge efficiency, efficacy, and lower costs.

1.7.2 REDUCTION IN HEALTHCARE COST

The costs pertaining to caring for health-related concerns are very expensive. These costs keep on growing across the board. Healthcare firms and practitioners can get detailed models for dropping patient recovery and risk costs using predictive and descriptive analytics. In addition to the benefits, AI and data analytics together can diminish no-show appointments, control the cost of supply chain management, and decrease numerous other kinds of fraud.

1.8 CONCLUSION

Proper management of the healthcare [17] data is the need of the hour, to use it properly. Data or essential information can be immediately accessed whenever required if and only if datasets are properly centralized by AI and data analytics. It additionally improves the efficiency and effectiveness of all prospects. Better data means a well-organized form of data. Properly organizing the data plays a vital role in better conclusions or analysis of a given set of data. It can be achieved with the help of AI and data analytics together. The main advantages of merging AI and data analytics in the healthcare sector are predictive modeling and reduction in healthcare costs. They both can lead the medical industry to great heights.

KEYWORDS

- **artificial intelligence**
- **data analytics**
- **e-commerce**
- **healthcare**
- **healthcare cost**
- **medical industry**
- **predictive modeling**
- **supply chain management**

REFERENCES

1. Yang, J. J., Li, J., Mulder, J., Wang, Y., Chen, S., Wu, H., Wang, Q., & Pan, H. (2015). Emerging information technologies for enhanced healthcare. *Computers in Industry, 69*, 3–11. doi: 10.1016/j.compind.2015.01.012.
2. Cortada, J. W., Gordon, D., & Lenihan, B. (2012). "The value of analytics in healthcare." *IBM Institute for Business Value IBM, Global Business Service* (2012).
3. Prokosch, H. U., & Ganslandt, T. (2009). Perspectives for medical informatics. *Methods of Information in Medicine, 48*, 38–44. doi: 10.3414/ME9132.
4. Simpao, A. F., Ahumada, L. M., Gálvez, J. A., & Rehman, M. A. (2014). A review of analytics and clinical informatics in health care. *Journal of Medical Systems, 38*, 45. doi: 10.1007/s10916-014-0045-x.
5. Dinov, I. D. (2016). Methodological challenges and analytic opportunities for modeling and interpreting Big Healthcare Data. *Gigascience, 5*, 12dnsdnsd12. doi: 10.1186/s13742-016-0117-6.

6. Chawla, N. V., & Davis, D. A. (2013). Bringing big data to personalized healthcare: A patient-centered framework. *Journal of General Internal Medicine, 28*, S660–S665. doi: 10.1007/s11606-013-2455-8.
7. Khalilia, M., Chakraborty, S., & Popescu, M. (2011). Predicting disease risks from highly imbalanced data using random forest. *BMC Medical Informatics and Decision Making, 11*, 51. doi: 10.1186/1472-6947-11-51.
8. Stamm, A. M., & Bettacchi, C. J. (2012). A comparison of 3 metrics to identify health care-associated infections. *American Journal of Infection Control, 40*, 688–691. doi: 10.1016/j.ajic.2012.01.033.
9. Dinov, I. D., Heavner, B., Tang, M., Glusman, G., Chard, K., Darcy, M., & Kesselman, C. (2016). Predictive big data analytics: A study of Parkinson's disease using large, complex, heterogeneous, incongruent, multi-source and incomplete observations. *PLoS ONE, 11*, e0157077. doi: 10.1371/journal.pone.0157077.
10. Mathias, J. S., Agrawal, A., Feinglass, J., Cooper, A. J., Baker, D. W., & Choudhary, A. (2013). Development of a 5-year life expectancy index in older adults using predictive mining of electronic health record data. *Journal of the American Medical Informatics Association, 20*, e118–e124. doi: 10.1136/amiajnl-2012-001360.
11. Sturgeon, L. P., Bragg-Underwood, D., Tonya, M., & Blankenship, D. (2016). Practice matters: Prevention and care of individuals with type 2 diabetes. *International Journal of Faith Community Nursing, 2*, 32–40.
12. National Center for Health Statistics (US), and National Center for Health Services Research. *Health, United States*. US Department of Health, Education, and Welfare, Public Health Service, Health Resources Administration, National Center for Health Statistics, 2012.
13. Angus, D. C., Barnato, A. E., Linde-Zwirble, W. T., Weissfeld, L. A., Watson, R. S., Rickert, T., & Rubenfeld, G. D. (2004). Use of intensive care at the end of life in the United States: An epidemiologic study. *Critical Care Medicine, 32*, 638–643. doi: 10.1097/01.CCM.0000114816.62331.08.
14. Saeed, M., Villarroel, M., Reisner, A. T., Clifford, G., Lehman, L. W., Moody, G., & Mark, R. G. (2011). Multiparameter Intelligent Monitoring in Intensive Care II (MIMIC-II): A public-access intensive care unit database. *Critical Care Medicine, 39*, 952–960. doi: 10.1097/CCM.0b013e31820a92c6.
15. Post, A. R., Kurc, T., Cholleti, S., Gao, J., Lin, 2., Bornstein, W., & Saltz, J. H. (2013). The Analytic Information Warehouse (AIW): A platform for analytics using electronic health record data. *Journal of Biomedical Informatics, 46*, 410–424. doi: 10.1016/j.jbi.2013.01.005.
16. Zhou, 2., Chen, S., Liu, B., Zhang, R., Wang, Y., Li, P., & Yan, 2. (2010). Development of traditional Chinese medicine clinical data warehouse for medical knowledge discovery and decision support. *Artificial Intelligence in Medicine, 48*, 139–152. doi: 10.1016/j.artmed.2009.07.012.
17. Zhang, Y., Qiu, M., Tsai, C. W., Hassan, M. M., & Alamri, A. (2015). Health-CPS: Healthcare cyber-physical system assisted by cloud and big data. *IEEE Systems Journal, 11*, 88–95. doi: 10.1109/JSYST.2015.2460747.
18. Pur, A., Bohanec, M., Lavrač, N., & Cestnik, B. (2010). Primary health-care network monitoring: A hierarchical resource allocation modeling approach. *International Journal of Health Planning and Management, 25*, 119–135. doi: 10.1002/hpm.1001.

19. Robinson, J. W. (2008). Regression tree boosting to adjust health care cost predictions for diagnostic mix. *Health Services Research, 43*, 755–772. doi: 10.1111/j.1475-6773.2007.00761. x.
20. Cercone, N., An, A., Li, J., Gu, Z., & An, A. (2011). Finding best evidence for evidence-based best practice recommendations in health care: The initial decision support system design. *Knowledge and Information Systems, 29*(1), 159–201. doi: 10.1007/s10115-011-0439-8.
21. Feldman, K., & Chawla, N. V. (2015). Does Medical School Training Relate to Practice? Evidence from Big Data. *Big Data, 3*, 103–113. doi: 10.1089/big.2014.0060.
22. Christodoulakis, A., Karanikas, H., Billiris, A., Thireos, E., & Pelekis, N. (2016). "Big data" in health care Assessment of the performance of Greek NHS hospitals using key performance and clinical workload indicators. *Archives of Hellenic Medicine, 33*, 489–497.
23. John, U., Hensel, E., Lüdemann, J., Piek, M., Sauer, S., Adam, C., & Greiser, E. (2001). Study of Health in Pomerania (SHIP): A health examination survey in an east German region: Objectives and design. *Sozial-und Präventivmedizin, 46*, 186–194. doi: 10.1007/BF01324255.
24. Milenkovic, M. J., Vukmirovic, A., & Milenkovic, D. (2019). Big data analytics in the health sector: Challenges and potentials. *Management: Journal of Sustainable Business and Management Solutions in Emerging Economies, 24*(1), 23–33.
25. Iyamu, T. (2020). A framework for selecting analytics tools to improve healthcare big data usefulness in developing countries. *South African Journal of Information Management, 22*(1), 1–9.
26. Poornima, S., & Pushpalatha, M. (2018). A survey of predictive analytics using big data with data mining. *International Journal of Bioinformatics Research and Applications, 14*(3), 269–282.
27. Pashazadeh, A., & Navimipour, N. J. (2018). Big data handling mechanisms in healthcare applications: A comprehensive and systematic literature review. *Journal of Biomedical Informatics, 82*, 47–62.
28. Sakr, S., & Elgammal, A. (2016). Towards a comprehensive data analytics framework for smart healthcare services. *Big Data Research, 4*, 44–58.
29. Singh, R. P., Javaid, M., Haleem, A., & Suman, R. (2020). Internet of things (IoT) applications to fight against COVID-19 pandemic. *Diabetes & Metabolic Syndrome: Clinical Research & Reviews, 14, 521*–524. doi: 10.1016/j.dsx.2020.04.040.
30. Vaishya, R., Javaid, M., Khan, I. H., & Haleem, A. (2020). Artificial intelligence (AI) applications for COVID-19 pandemic. *Diabetes & Metabolic Syndrome: Clinical Research & Reviews, 14, 337–339.* doi: 10.1016/j.dsx.2020.04.032.

CHAPTER 2

Biomimetics and Mind-Machine Interface: The Human Brain as a Quantum Computer

ARKAJIT BHATTACHARYA[1] and A. B. BHATTACHARYA[2]

[1]*Indian Institute of Engineering Science and Technology, Institute Hospital Unit, Shibpur, Howrah, West Bengal, India*

[2]*Brainware University, Barasat, Kolkata, West Bengal, India*

ABSTRACT

In theory, biomimicry can be used in a number of developing industries. The complexity of biological systems results in a very high number of visible traits. Biomimetic applications can be seen at different phases of technological development in a wide range of application domains. In recent years, a variety of tools have been created to communicate with neurons and networks. Experiments have been developed to create robotic gadgets and problem-solving networks using cutting-edge technology. Early in 2017, a competent team of computer programmers and neuroscientists worked together to advance our understanding of the human mind. A person's peripheral nerves carry bundles of fibers that allow nerve cells to communicate with various areas of the hand. Three nerves are present in the human hand, and there are numerous ways to reestablish touch using these nerves. A system that takes the time-varying force signal and its derivatives should be ready in order to duplicate any signal that has peripheral feedback. This enhances the signal's contact timing—that is, the interval between when it maintains and loses touch with the object.

Data-Driven Analytics for Healthcare: Artificial Intelligence and Machine Learning for Medical Diagnostics.
Meghna Sharma, Priyanka Vashisht, A. V. Senthil Kumar, Chitra Singh, and Abdelmalek Amine (Eds.)

Modern simulation models have been created to simulate several facets of transduction. An arbitrary space-time simulation is produced as a result of the skin mechanics model, which models the mechanical bending of the skin. These virtual touch models on computers allow for artificial touch sensitivity. As a non-invasive brain-computer interface (BCI), magnetoencephalography (MEG) and functional magnetic resonance imaging (fMRI) have been employed with convenience. Microtubules are an essential part of the neural scaffolding and are crucial in both biology and neuroscience. Consciousness is made of information contained in microtubules. According to the theory of quantum consciousness, the brain functions like a quantum computer, and consciousness is the state of the brain's quantum information. The fundamental theories and numerous uses of these compounds were thoroughly covered in this chapter.

2.1 INTRODUCTION

Today's quick advancements in health science and related technology have helped people live longer and conquer many complex ailments [1]. Nevertheless, over time, rising pollution and environmental deterioration have negatively impacted human existence. It is true that engineers and scientists work hard to develop new goods that will make our lives better. The right method was not always correctly identified since a very clear answer to resource shortages and survival difficulties was not always given the highest priority. Biomimetics might be an emerging strategy to deal with these problems. Despite the fact that biomimetics is not a recent subject or trend, careful adoption of new technologies during the past 20 years has shown much higher success rates. It is heartening that recently; humanity has allowed substantial advancements in brain-computer interface and biomimetic technology [2]. This chapter has been devoted to discussing biomimetics, including their current uses and anticipated future applications. The terms used in the research field that are pertinent to the case are highlighted and defined.

2.1.1 NEURAL CELLS

The basic building blocks of the nervous system and the brain are known as neurons. The cells are employed to take sensory information from the outside world and use that information to provide motor instructions to our muscles. Its function is to transform and relay electrical signals between devices. In nerve tissue, there are just two main cells. While the other cell is referred to as a neuroglia (which means nerve glue), the neuron is the "conducting" cell that transmits impulses. In order to transport information between the brain and the nervous system, as well as between different parts of the brain, neurons use both electrical and chemical signals. This allows neurons to govern and coordinate many bodily functions.

2.1.2 NEURAL TISSUE

Also known as nervous tissue, neural tissue is the basic tissue that makes up the neurological system and regulates bodily function. The spinal cord, nerves, and brain all include this tissue. In addition to playing a crucial part in memory, logic, and emotions, it is in charge of causing muscular contraction. The two primary cells that make up the nervous tissue are the neurons and the neuroglia. Neurons benefit from the support provided by unique non-conductive forms of "connective tissue" called neuroglia.

2.1.3 BUILDING PROBLEM-SOLVING

Problem-solving develops tools for applying mathematical knowledge to solve real-world problems. Problem-solving is enjoyable. Organizational problems are solved by going methodically through each stage and identifying an appropriate solution. The problem-solving approach is a technique that can be utilized for better understanding the problems and developing optimal solutions in a more innovative way.

2.1.4 ROBOTIC APPARELS

It is an interdisciplinary area of computer science and engineering that deals with the creation, maintenance, and use of robots, which are machines that can be programmed by computers to do a complex series of tasks automatically. Robots are controlled either internally by the system or externally by a control device. Robotics is a branch of engineering that deals with building machines that can work on their own.

2.1.5 THE HUMAN MIND

It is a collection of faculties that includes sensation, will, memory, imagination, and thought. Billions of nerve cells in the human brain are made up of ideas and images in the mind. The invisible energy of thought is a sophisticated neurological system that links the brain to the rest of the body. About 23 watts is the maximum amount of energy that our brains can produce. The pathways in the brain are maintained by getting enough sleep, and it may also promote the accumulation of a protein associated with Alzheimer's disease.

2.1.6 PERIPHERAL NERVES OF THE HUMAN BODY

These nerves are located apart from the brain and spinal cord. They aid in the communication of information between the brain and the body as a whole. The autonomic nervous system regulates glands and bodily processes. Accidental injuries, diabetes, Guillain-Barre syndrome, and carpal tunnel syndrome can all cause damage to peripheral nerves.

2.1.7 SIGNALING

In biochemistry, the term "signaling" refers to the transmission of a biochemical signal. Juxtacrine signaling, another name for direct signaling, is a term used to describe communication between cells that are in close proximity to one another. Autocrine signaling, on the other hand, occurs when a ligand works on the same cell to release it. Cell signaling occurs in three stages: reception, where the signal molecule attaches to the receptor; transduction, where the chemical signal causes a string of enzyme activations; and response, which describes the physiological reactions that follow.

2.1.8 TRANSDUCTION

The process by which a virus spreads genetic material from one bacterium to another is known as transduction. Bacteriophages, which are viruses, infect bacterial cells and use them as hosts to manufacture further viruses.

The binding of an extracellular messenger to a cell surface receptor during signal transduction causes the receptor to respond to the information being received. In genetic engineering, the transduction procedure is typically used to transfer foreign DNA into the host cell.

2.1.9 SKIN MECHANICS

The skin is the biggest organ in the body and is made of flexible material. An internal organ is made up of its derivatives, including hair, nails, perspiration, and sebaceous glands. Melanin, a pigment produced by certain skin cells, is what gives skin its color. The skin shields the body from environmental dangers like temperature, toxins, and bacteria. Skin cells are made of keratin, a protein found in skin cells, which binds to other proteins to form this layer. The multilayered mechanical characteristics of human skin are crucial.

2.1.10 TACTILE SENSATION

The tactile sense enables us to remain aware of our surroundings. The human sense of touch is connected to a variety of skin receptors that can pick up signals concerning pressure, temperature, vibration, texture, pain, and limb position and transmit them to the brain via our neurological system.

2.1.11 MAGNETOENCEPHALOGRAPHY (MEG)

This non-invasive medical test assesses the magnetic fields produced by electrical currents in the brain. It pinpoints the precise site of the epileptic seizures' origin and maps brain function. MEG tests are conducted in a magnetically shielded environment. Because MEG offers a higher temporal resolution than fMRI, it is possible to monitor brain activity more precisely at certain times.

2.1.12 FUNCTIONAL MAGNETIC RESONANCE IMAGING (FMRI)

It is extremely successful in safely and non-invasively detecting brain activity. It measures minute variations in blood flow in an active area of the brain using MR imaging. The primary benefit of fMRI is that it does not use radiation, unlike computed tomography (CT) and positron emission tomography (PET), which both involve radiation. When used properly, fMRI poses essentially no hazards.

2.1.13 BRAIN-COMPUTER INTERFACE (BCI)

It is a computer system that collects brain signals, analyzes them, and transforms them into instructions that may be sent to an output device to carry out a desired activity. BCI is a technology for assisting, adapting, and healing that tracks brain activity and modifies signal characteristics to reflect commands given to any device. The method uses electrophysiological impulses to directly control the computer cursor. Without using the typical neuromuscular routes, the system aids in communication with the outside world. BCIs come in two varieties: non-invasive and invasive.

2.1.14 MICROTUBULES

Microtubules are proteins that give cells structural support. They are necessary for cell division, which involves the movement of chromosomes to opposite ends of the cell. They can be present in all eukaryotic cells and are the basic building blocks of the cytoskeleton. Together, alpha- and beta-tubulin subunits form microtubules. The microtubule network is recognized for its major function in controlling cell motility and growth, as well as for modulating basic cellular functions through signaling.

2.1.15 QUANTUM CONSCIOUSNESS

Quantum consciousness, also known as quantum mind, emphasizes how essential quantum-mechanical phenomena, such as entanglement and superposition, are to the functioning of the brain and the explanation of consciousness. Consciousness in the brain and nonlocal properties are related via the quantum soul. The fact that the human brain is made up of atoms that obey quantum physics laws suggests that our thoughts are connected to a cosmic mind.

2.2 BIOMIMETICS

The Greek words bios (life) and mimesis (to copy), together form the phrase "biomimetic." Its definition, however, is different. First and foremost, biomimetics is a creative way to mimic nature in order to enhance people's lives. In the fields of architecture, chemistry, biology, engineering, medicine, and biomedical engineering, biomimetics is used to improve general industry and human comfort.

In different regions of the world, biomimetics has been referred to by different names, such as smart materials in the USA and intellectual structure in Japan. As a result of resource exploitation and industrialization, humans have significantly altered nature. However, this situation can be avoided with the right application of biomimetics. As shown in Figure 2.1, biomimetics can produce new products that are suitably designed to play a significant role in general industry and to provide human convenience in various fields such as architecture, biology, chemistry, medicine, and primarily biomedical engineering. Its applications are endless since this symbiotic relationship is crucial to the coexistence of man and nature. Understanding the areas with suitable execution for each of them is thus always advised [3, 4].

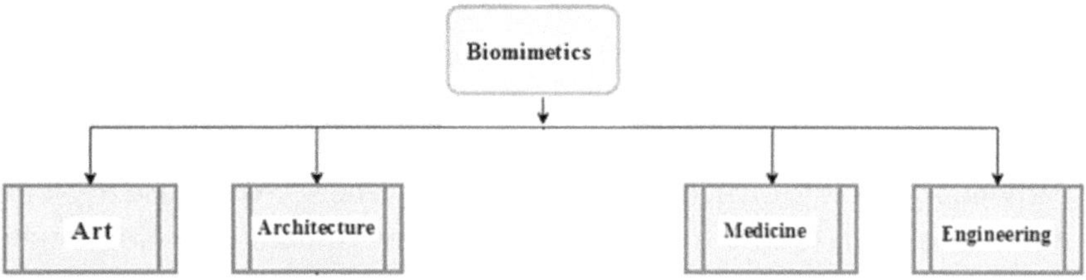

FIGURE 2.1 Areas of applications in biomimetics.

2.2.1 HISTORIES OF DEVELOPMENT

The subject of applied science known as biomimetics has a lengthy history. The work of Leonardo da Vinci (1452–1519), who created a flying contraption after watching a flying bird, is a very good example of biomimicry [5]. In order to counter Japanese raiders during invasions, General Yi Sun-sin in the Far East created a warship model (the turtle ship) like a turtle. The Wright brothers (1867–1948) first achieved success with a motorized airplane in 1903, noting eagle wings [6, 7]. Schmitt's adoption of the term "biomimetic" in 1957 marked a significant advancement in both biology and technology [8]. The term "biomimicry" was first used in an article by NASA's Jack E. Steele in 1969. In 1997, Janine M. Benyus wrote a book on the subject, solidifying its position as the main route for technological advancement. Instead of using science as a raw material, she placed an emphasis on using it as the foundation of goods [9]. Soon after, a group of researchers, artists, engineers, scientists, business executives, and stakeholders were brought together by the concepts of biomimicry and biomimetics.

2.2.2 TECHNIQUES IMPLEMENTED FOR BIOMIMETICS

The basic research methodology for biomimetics consists of six parts. These procedures can be used to apply biomimetics to a range of designs, goods, and services in various industries [10]. In serious study, rather than applying for simple design consideration, the functional possibilities of biologically inspired design have taken an essential part in developing the creative design idea with a view to improving convenience for human everyday life. Utilizing database compilation, a thorough understanding and application of many types of materials must be acquired. The surface structure typically influences the relationship between structure and function. SEM is a technology that can be used to accomplish this. The fine structures produced are crucial to the creature, and this is seen to be the beginning of biomimicry. Finding the relationship between the function of nano- and micro-structures and the organism and the environment is a particularly notable difficulty in the field [10]. The second phase in biomimetic research is to find significant examples by combining biology, material science, and natural history. The use of numerous environmental and action systems used by organisms, as well as their energy-saving design, might be thought of as the next research area. A good illustration of this is an anti-reflective coating that was modeled after 200 nm patterns that deflect light rays visible to moth eyes [11–13]. These biomimetic materials' nature is based on how hierarchical structures act for remodeling and improved utilization. For applications with various limits, combining recently found materials with biomimetic research can be regarded as a significant insight [9, 10]. The new material's morphological and functional advantages must be emphasized. Although several areas of research are actively being pursued, nothing has been accomplished thus far. The definition of biological material structures and the use of their associated functions is a major source of inspiration for the creation of novel materials. New, better materials can be created using current understanding of the structure and purpose of established materials. Then, in order to create new utilities for improving human existence, these are integrated with modern developments in chemistry, medicine, and nanotechnology.

2.3 BIOMIMETIC ROBOTS

Recently, biomimetic technology has been applied to a variety of industries, including design, agriculture, material science, chemistry, and, most notably, medical. Additionally, biomimetic robots were attempted to be applied in a new field [14, 15].

For RHex to have robotic legs to get over the wheel restriction, a cockroach leg mechanism was discovered [16]. To replicate the bones and joints of the elephant trunk and stomach, other robotic arms have been created [17]. Using the tiny hairs on a gecko's soles, scientists created an iRobot that was sensitive to pressure and capable of strong dry adhesion.

2.4 BIOMIMETICS APPLIED TO HEALTH SCIENCE AND BIOMEDICAL ENGINEERING

In essence, biomimetics is a method for solving the issues with theory-development technology in the biological sciences. It works with nature and natural occurrences to comprehend the fundamentals of their underlying mechanisms and apply notions that can be helpful to science, technology, and medicine. With the help of various handy items, biomimetics, whose designs are inspired by living things, has made people's lives better. The treatment of numerous complicated disorders in addition to physical traumas has a stronger impact on the merger of medicine, science, and biomedical technology. Tissue engineering and regenerative medicine are currently regarded as two very promising topics. The ideas of biomimetics used in biomedical engineering are borrowed from a variety of sources, such as the Koran, the yearly growth of a lizard's tail, a spider's ability to regenerate, etc. A biocompatible medical dressing that can be used in a universal healthcare system (U-health) that is compatible with human tissue serves as a good illustration. It delivers precise real-time reports on the state of disease or healing. Signal detection can be accomplished using a biocompatible tape or a temporary medical bandage. Heart attacks or myocardial infarctions that cannot be identified or tracked by existing medical instruments can be successfully monitored with the help of these signals. This style of clothes would be less irritating and would be suited for human skin. Gecko leg hairs can provide this function [18].

To address complex issues, biomimetics blends biology and other technologies. Understanding materials and their structures through the use of nanotechnology can help expand our understanding of protein structure, which has the potential to be employed in a number of novel applications [19]. In order to employ hybrid compounds as a model for controlling biological processes in tissue engineering, natural hybrid compounds have been created. To explain their structural complexity, structural biomaterials like bone and nacre are organized hierarchically. Developments of morphological structures of inorganic-organic hybrid materials are vital to replicate biological and structural formations. As native tissue architecture, fibrous scaffolds with several functions are created. These offer a great deal of potential for bone regeneration. Biomimicking scaffold materials show higher efficacy for tissue repair and regeneration [20]. Biomimetics is currently being quickly incorporated into biomedical engineering. An example of how biomimetics and bioengineering can be combined to generate a novel material that may be used in medical operations is the development of syringe needles that don't hurt.

The structure of the mosquito's mouth canal, which can draw blood from the host animal with the least amount of nerve discomfort, was also modeled by the researchers. For diabetics and during surgery to assist people in overcoming their needle phobia, this kind of needle is helpful. To make these needles safer and more useful than conventional micro-silicon needles, makers use polylactic acid, a biodegradable polymer. These needles have an angular shape as a result of the varied properties of cellular microenvironments. Cellular characteristics are explored using biomimetic platforms for analytical reasons, which deliver living models of complicated environments [21–23]. The interactions between cells in lymph nodes, where two different types of cells dynamically communicate through immunological signals, are mimicked by researchers working on this subject using specific engineering techniques. Researchers who create biomimetic cell environments can find practical answers to the interaction between cells and the microenvironment around them as microenvironments advance.

2.4.1 BRAIN-COMPUTER INTERFACES (BCI)

Through gesture, speech, written communication, social connection, or communication, one is able to express expectations, feelings, and creative ideas. People who have locked-in syndrome are unable to interact or express their emotions. Cerebral palsy, brain stem stroke, amyotrophic lateral sclerosis (ALS), multiple sclerosis, and spinal cord injury are the main causes of locked-in syndrome [24]. The brain-computer interface provides an alternate means of communicating using fundamental communication abilities. The BCI concept underpins this technology, and users must generate a variety of brain waves in order to interpret those waves into instructions for the apparatus [25]. Figure 2.2 depicts the general design of brain-computer interfaces.

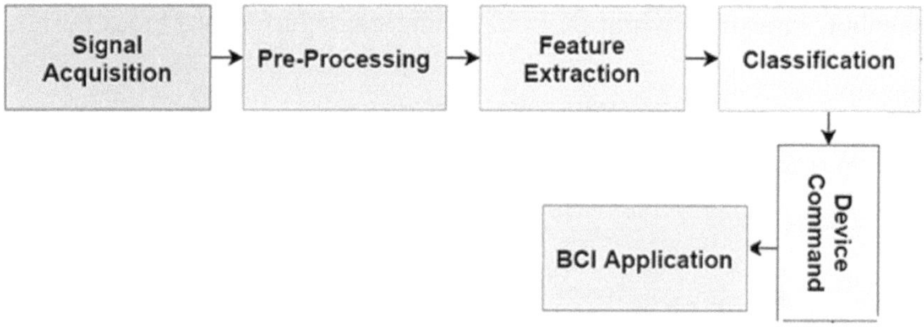

FIGURE 2.2 The general architecture of a brain-computer interfacing.

The development of technology began with aids intended solely for medicinal use. It has, however, also been frequently used for non-medical purposes. There is currently a lengthy list of particular medical applications, such as wheelchair control [26, 27], biometrics [28, 29], BCI mobile robot [30], and emotion recognition utilizing Electroencephalogram (EEG) [31]. Applications relating to EEG-based BCI systems were focused on EEG control signals and their classifications [32, 33]. EEG control signals, classification techniques, their precision, and characteristics were examined by Lotte et al. [34–36]. An overview of EEG, functional transcranial Doppler (fTCD), and near-infrared spectroscopy (NIRS)-based hybrid BCI was published [37], with an emphasis on the EEG control signal, experiment protocol, signal processing techniques, and system evaluation, as well as future directions for EEG-based BCI research. Traditional BCI methods have only ever used brain signals to generate output. However, it was shown that the fundamental properties of brain signals can differ between individuals. In reality, from trial to trial, the characteristics of the same object could occasionally change. Analysis of specific features or operations might occasionally result in the omission of crucial data. Due to these difficulties, machine learning is a good choice for signal categorization and discrimination. Machine learning is utilized in many different domains of application to address problems of all kinds, and it has also been successful in addressing problems relating to BCI signals. Machine learning techniques might significantly improve decoding precision. The BCI system records and examines a number of additional signals in order to strengthen the system's robustness, increase data transmission, and shorten training time. To merge complementary signals, these systems employ machine learning algorithms and data fusion techniques. Figure 2.3 illustrates this method, known as hybrid BCI [38], using a straightforward block design.

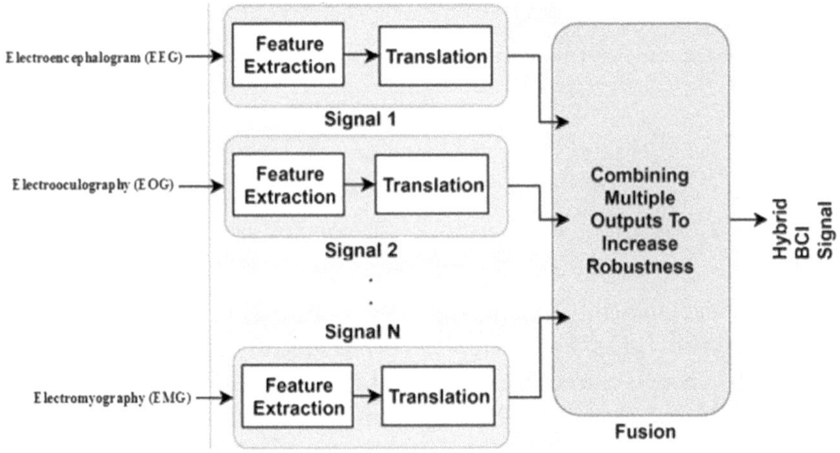

FIGURE 2.3 A simple block diagram of hybrid BCI.

Source: Adapted from Ref. [38].

2.4.2 BCI SYSTEM USED FOR PHYSIOLOGIC SIGNALS

Any brain signal may theoretically be utilized to power a BCI device. The most often used signals are the electrical signals, which mostly come from polarity changes in the postsynaptic membranes of neurons brought on by the activation of voltage or ion channels. These signals make up a substantial portion of Hans Berger's scalp EEG observation [39]. BCI initially made use of scalp-recorded EEG signals. They had the benefit of being secure, simple, and affordable to get, but they have a substantial drawback in that they lost a lot of data due to the electrical signals in scalp recordings being significantly attenuated as they passed through the skull and scalp [40]. In order to record both local field potentials and action potentials of specific neurons, tiny intra-cortical microarrays were implanted in the brain. These implants have the drawbacks of being invasive, having a small recording area, and having long-term functional stability of the recording electrodes. Another option for recording brain signals is using BCIs based on electrocorticography (ECoG). With this method, intra-parenchymal [41, 42] or intra-ventricular [43] recordings can be made of the signals obtained from grid or strip electrodes placed on the cortex's surface. These electrode arrays, like intra-cortical microarrays, record intra-cranially from greater brain regions, but they again have the drawback of requiring neurosurgical implantation for the electrodes. The best option for the individual is picked after weighing the benefits and drawbacks of different approaches. Modern methods for recording brain signals for BCI control now include high-resolution functional neuroimaging. In essence, magnetoencephalography (MEG) measures the fields created by electric currents traveling in the direction of pyramidal cell axons. Blood oxygenation in a brain region is detected using functional magnetic resonance imaging (fMRI) and functional near-infrared imaging (fNIR), both of which correlate with neuronal activity. Lee et al. [44] demonstrated that the only way a real-time fMRI-based BCI could be used to control a robotic arm was through the user's thoughts. In this context, it should be noted that MEG and fMRI are quite costly and sophisticated, whereas fMRI and fNIR have rather slow response times.

2.5 MICROTUBULE: INTERPLAY OF BIOCHEMISTRY AND HEALTH SCIENCE

The polarized hollow cylinders known as microtubules, which are made of the proteins alpha- and beta-tubulin, are thought to control the direction of cell migration [45–50]. These are characterized by a continuous cycle of growing and contracting, which is called dynamic instability [51–54] and play a significant role in cellular processes [55]. Dynamic instability is the main characteristic that defines microtubules. They have significant functions in the kidney, brain, and cell lines, among other cell populations. Tubulin is a flexible protein that has undergone a great deal of post-translational modification. Some of them have been studied in brain tissue. It has been found that the mutant tubulin assembles inside a cell, as shown in Figure 2.4 [56–60]. Dynamic instability is the term used to describe how microtubules typically proceed through cycles of polymerization and depolymerization. However, it has been discovered that some microtubule subpopulations are stabilized. Microtubule-associated proteins (MAPs), formins, and microtubule plus-end transport proteins (+TIPs) promote this process, which requires coating beta-tubulin monomers with guanosine triphosphate (GTP). As a result of this stabilization, microtubules undergo post-translational modifications such as acetylation and detyrosination.

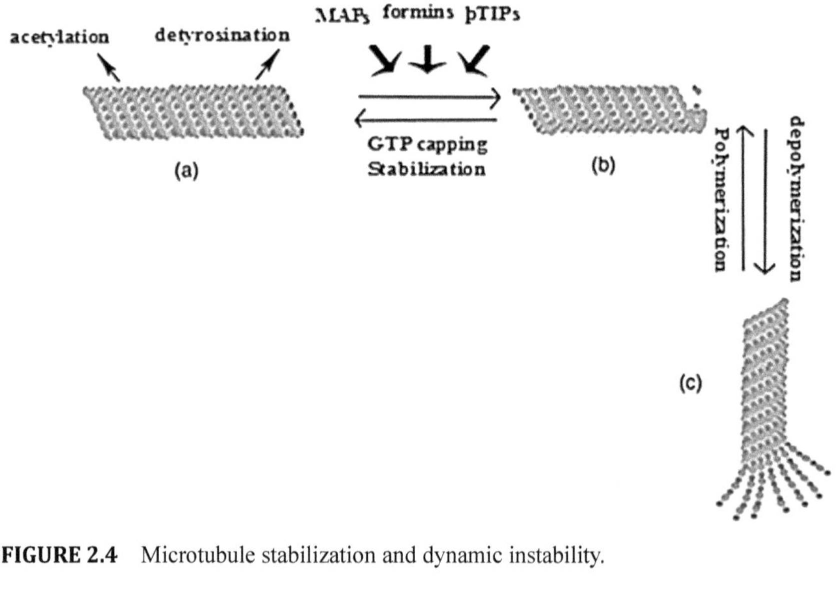

FIGURE 2.4 Microtubule stabilization and dynamic instability.

Brain development and regeneration are among the modifications brought on by these post-translational modifications [61, 62].

2.6 CONCLUSION

The subjects of biomimetics have been produced even without the assistance of traditional research [63]. Humanity has significantly increased progress, but this industrialization has also put our survival in danger and polluted the environment. Therefore, it is vital that alternative methods for technical materials, goods and services be found. Perhaps biomimicry is viewed as a very effective strategy for the advancement of civilization, overcoming the risks of resource scarcity and environmental damage on a big scale. The best method to coexist with nature is seen to be through biomimicry. The surface structures of animals, plants, and insects have demonstrated long-term evolution. Beginning as a straightforward replication of living things, biomimetics gradually advanced through integration. Collaborations with contemporary science and technology can aid our search for novel materials. This may show how to mix microstructures, uses, and even different production techniques.

As technology develops, we can anticipate seeing things that are more environmentally friendly and biodegradable being produced. How much we can use nature will determine how creative we can be with new materials. BCI systems can employ everything from wheelchairs to robotic arms and utilize a range of brain signals and signal processing algorithms. Patients with severe disabilities can use a BCI for everyday control and rudimentary communication. In the near future, BCIs may develop into a significant new communication and control tool for both people with impairments and the general public with improved clinical validation. Microtubules, a crucial component of the cellular cytoskeleton, are linked to brain-computer interfaces because they play a significant part in biomimetics. We are awaiting additional research to confirm the highly interacting nature of the cell-to-cytoskeletal network.

ACKNOWLEDGMENTS

One of the authors (Dr. Arkajit Bhattacharya) would like to express his sincere thanks to the Director, of the Indian Institute of Engineering and Technology (Shibpur, Howrah) for providing the research facility. The corresponding author of the chapter (Prof. A. B. Bhattacharya) is thankful to the Chancellor of Brainware University for his encouragement and support.

KEYWORDS

- **biomimetics**
- **computational models**
- **guanosine triphosphate**
- **microtubule-associated proteins**
- **microtubules**
- **neuroscience**
- **quantum consciousness**

REFERENCES

1. Rashid, M., Sulaiman, N., Abdul Majeed, A. P. P., Musa, R. M., Ab. Nasir, A. F., Bari, B. S., & Khatun, S. (2020). Current status, challenges, and possible solutions of EEG-based brain-computer interface: A comprehensive review. *Frontiers in Neurorobotics, 14*, 25. doi: 10.3389/fnbot.2020.00025.
2. Bhattacharya, A. B., & Sen, P. (2018). *Brain Computer Interfacing Brain Computer Interface Technology & its Modern Applications*. LAP Lambert, Germany. ISBN 978-613-9-85478-3. pp. 1–324, 2018, LAP Lambert Academic Publishing, International Book Market Service Ltd.
3. Hwang, J., Jeong, Y., Park, J. M., Lee, K. H., Hong, J. W., & Choi, J. (2015). Biomimetics: Forecasting the future of science, engineering, and medicine. *International Journal of Nanomedicine, 10*, 5701–5713. doi: 10.2147/IJN.S83642.
4. Hargroves, K., & Smith, M. (2006). Innovation inspired by nature: Biomimicry. *ECOS, 129*, 27–29.
5. Vincent, J. F., Bogatyreva, O. A., Bogatyrev, N. R., Bowyer, A., & Pahl, A.-K. (2006). Biomimetics: Its practice and theory. *Journal of the Royal Society Interface, 3*(9), 471–482.
6. Freedman, R. (1991). *The Wright Brothers: How They Invented the Airplane*. New York: Holiday House. ISBN 13- 978–0823410828, Publisher: Holiday House, Publication Date: 1 January 1991.
7. Jakab, P. L. (1990). *Visions of a Flying Machine: Wright Brothers and the Process of Invention [Exhibition catalog]* Washington, D.C.: Smithsonian Institution Press, "https://research.si.edu/publication-details/?id=118026." Type: exhibition_catalog.
8. Schmitt, O. H. (1969). Some interesting and useful biomimetic transforms. Third International Biophysics Congress of the International Union for Pure and Applied Biophysics, Cambridge, 1969, p. 297.
9. Benyus, J. M. (2009). Biomimicry, Innovation Inspired by Nature, Harper Collins e-Books, Adobe Digital Edition. June 2009. ISBN 978–0-06–195892–2.

10. Shimomura, M. (2010). The new trends in next-generation biomimetics material technology: Learning from biodiversity. *Science and Technology Trends Quarterly Review, 37*, 53–75.
11. Goel, A. K., McAdams, D. A., & Stone, R. B. (Eds.). (2013). The AskNature Database: Enabling Solutions in Biomimetic Design Biologically Inspired Design. Vol. 2013. Springer; p. 20.
12. Lee, D. W., & Graham, R. (1986). Leaf optical properties of rainforest sun and extreme shade plants. *American Journal of Botany, 73*, 1100–1108.
13. Gabriel, C. T., Haskell, J., & Sethi, S. (2001). Sacrificial multilayer anti-reflective coating for MOS gate formation. Google Patents; 2001.
14. Witte, H., Hoffmann, H., Hackert, R., Schilling, C., Fischer, M. S., & Preuschoft, H. (2004). Biomimetic robotics should be based on functional morphology. *Journal of Anatomy, 204*(5), 331–342.
15. Boxerbaum, A. S., Shaw, K. M., Chiel, H. J., & Quinn, R. D. (2012). Continuous wave peristaltic motion in a robot. *International Journal of Robotics Research, 31*(3), 302–318.
16. Altendorfer, R., Moore, N., Komsuoglu, H., et al. (2001). RHex: A biologically inspired hexapod runner. *Autonomous Robots, 11*(3), 207–213.
17. Wright, C., Johnson, A., Peck, A., et al. (2007). Design of a modular snake robot. Paper presented at: *IEEE/RSJ International Conference on Intelligent Robots and Systems, 2007*. IROS 2007.
18. Mahan, G. D. (2014). Amorphous Solid. School & Library Products; 2014.
19. Gong, Y. K., & Winnik, F. M. (2012). Strategies in biomimetic surface engineering of nanoparticles for biomedical applications. *Nanoscale, 4*(2), 360–368.
20. Bao, M., Lou, X., Zhou, Q., Dong, W., Yuan, H., & Zhang, Y. (2014). Electrospun biomimetic fibrous scaffold from shape memory polymer of PDLLA-co-TMC for bone tissue engineering. *ACS Applied Materials & Interfaces, 6*(4), 2611–2621.
21. Kim, Y. C., Park, J. H., & Prausnitz, M. R. (2012). Microneedles for drug and vaccine delivery. *Advanced Drug Delivery Reviews, 64*(14), 1547–1568. doi: 10.1016/j.addr.2012.04.005.
22. Izumi, H., Suzuki, M., Aoyagi, S., & Kanzaki, T. (2011). Realistic imitation of mosquito's proboscis: Electrochemically etched sharp and jagged needles and their cooperative inserting motion. *Sensors and Actuators A: Physical, 165*(1), 115–123. doi: 10.1016/j.sna.2010.10.011.
23. Choi, J., Hwang, M. P., Lee, J. W., & Lee, K. H. (2014). A glimpse into the interactions of cells in a microenvironment: The modulation of T cells by mesenchymal stem cells. *International Journal of Nanomedicine, 9*(suppl 1), 127. doi: 10.2147/IJN.S58058.
24. Holz, E. M., Höhne, J., Staiger-Sälzer, P., Tangermann, M., & Kübler, A. (2013). Brain-computer interface-controlled gaming: Evaluation of usability by severely motor restricted end-users. *Artificial Intelligence in Medicine, 59*(2), 111–120. doi: 10.1016/j.artmed.2013.08.001.
25. Volosyak, I., Gembler, F., & Stawicki, P. (2017). Age-related differences in SSVEP-based BCI performance. *Neurocomputing, 250*, 57–64. doi: 10.1016/j.neucom.2016.08.121.

26. Fernández-Rodríguez, Á., Velasco-Álvarez, F., & Ron-Angevin, R. (2016). Review of real brain-controlled wheelchairs. *Journal of Neural Engineering, 13*(6), 061001. doi: 10.1088/1741-2560/13/6/061001.
27. Al-qaysi, Z. T., Zaidan, B. B., Zaidan, A. A., & Suzani, M. S. (2018). A review of disability EEG-based wheelchair control system: Coherent taxonomy, open challenges and recommendations. *Computer Methods and Programs in Biomedicine, 164*, 221–237. doi: 10.1016/j.cmpb.2018.06.012.
28. Del Pozo-Banos, M., Alonso, J. B., Ticay-Rivas, J. R., & Travieso, C. M. (2014). Electroencephalogram subject identification: A review. *Expert Systems with Applications, 41*(15), 6537–6554. doi: 10.1016/j.eswa.2014.05.013.
29. Alariki, A. A., Ibrahimi, A. W., Wardak, M., & Wall, J. (2018). A review study of brain activity-based biometric authentication. *Journal of Computer Science, 14*(2), 173–181. doi: 10.3844/jcssp.2018.173.181.
30. Bi, L., Fan, X.-A., & Liu, Y. (2013). EEG-based brain-controlled mobile robots: A survey. *IEEE Transactions on Human-Machine Systems, 43*(2), 161–176. doi: 10.1109/TSMCC.2012.2219046.
31. Al-Nafjan, A., Hosny, M., Al-Ohali, Y., & Al-Wabil, A. (2017). Review and classification of emotion recognition based on EEG brain-computer interface system research: A systematic review. *Applied Sciences, 7*(12), 1239. doi: 10.3390/app7121239.
32. Ramadan, R. A., & Vasilakos, A. V. (2017). Brain computer interface: Control signals review. *Neurocomputing, 223*, 26–44. doi: 10.1016/j.neucom.2016.10.024.
33. Hwang, H. J., Kim, S., Choi, S., & Im, C. H. (2013). EEG-based brain-computer interfaces: A thorough literature survey. *International Journal of Human-Computer Interaction, 29*(12), 814–826. doi: 10.1080/10447318.2013.780869.
34. Lotte, F., Bougrain, L., Cichocki, A., Clerc, M., Congedo, M., Rakotomamonjy, A., et al. (2018). A review of classification algorithms for EEG-based brain-computer interfaces: A 10-year update. *Journal of Neural Engineering, 15*(3), 031005. doi: 10.1088/1741-2552/aab2f2.
35. Lotte, F., Bougrain, L., & Clerc, M. (2015). Electroencephalography (EEG)-based brain-computer interfaces. In J. Webster (Ed.), *Wiley Encyclopedia of Electrical and Electronics Engineering* (pp. 1–20). John Wiley and Sons, Inc. doi: 10.1002/047134608X.W8278.
36. Lotte, F., Congedo, M., Lécuyer, A., Lamarche, F., & Arnaldi, B. (2007). A review of classification algorithms for EEG-based brain–computer interfaces. *Journal of Neural Engineering, 4*(2), R1–R13. doi: 10.1088/1741-2560/4/2/R01.
37. Banville, H., & Falk, T. H. (2016). Recent advances and open challenges in hybrid brain-computer interfacing: A technological review of non-invasive human research. *Brain-Computer Interfaces, 3*(1), 9–46. doi: 10.1080/2326263X.2015.1134958.
38. Chamola, V., Vineet, A., Nayyar, A., & Hossain, E. (2020). Brain-computer interface-based humanoid control: A review. *Sensors, 20*(13), 3620. doi: 10.3390/s20133620.
39. Berger, H. (1929). Über das Electrenkephalogramm des Menschen. *Archiv für Psychiatrie und Nervenkrankheiten, 87*, 527–570.
40. Akhtari, M., Bryant, H. C., Mamelak, A. N., et al. (2000). Conductivities of three-layer human skull. *Brain Topography, 13*(1), 29–42.

41. Krusienski, D. J., & Shih, J. J. (2011). Control of a brain-computer interface using stereotactic depth electrodes in and adjacent to the hippocampus. *Journal of Neural Engineering, 8*(2), 025006. doi: 10.1088/1741-2560/8/2/025006.
42. Krusienski, D. J., & Shih, J. J. (2011). Control of a visual keyboard using an electrocorticographic brain-computer interface. *Neurorehabilitation and Neural Repair, 25*(4), 323–331. doi: 10.1177/1545968311401621.
43. Shih, J. J., & Krusienski, D. J. (2012). Signals from intraventricular depth electrodes can control a brain-computer interface. *Journal of Neuroscience Methods, 203*(2), 311–314. doi: 10.1016/j.jneumeth.2011.09.027.
44. Lee, J. H., Ryu, J., Jolesz, F. A., Cho, Z. H., & Yoo, S. S. (2009). Brain-machine interface via real-time fMRI: Preliminary study on thought-controlled robotic arm. *Neuroscience Letters, 450*(1), 1–6. doi: 10.1016/j.neulet.2008.11.034.
45. Adams Jr., G., Zhou, J., Wang, W., Wu, H., Quan, J., Liu, Y., & Yao, X. (2016). The microtubule plus end tracking protein TIP150 interacts with cortactin to steer directional cell migration. *Journal of Biological Chemistry, 291*(39), 20692–20706. doi: 10.1074/jbc.M116.734343.
46. Barth, A. I., Caro-Gonzalez, H. Y., & Nelson, W. J. (2008). Role of adenomatous polyposis coli (APC) and microtubules in directional cell migration and neuronal polarization. *Seminars in Cell & Developmental Biology, 19*(3), 245–251. doi: 10.1016/j.semcdb.2008.01.001.
47. Cao, D., Su, Z., Wang, W., Wu, H., Liu, X., Akram, S., & Yao, X. (2015). Signaling scaffold protein IQGAP1 interacts with microtubule plus-end tracking protein SKAP and links dynamic microtubule plus-end to steer cell migration. *Journal of Biological Chemistry, 290*(39), 23766–23780. doi: 10.1074/jbc.M115.669424.
48. Francis, R., Xu, X., Park, H., Wei, C. J., Chang, S., Chatterjee, B., & Lo, C. (2011). Connexin43 modulates cell polarity and directional cell migration by regulating microtubule dynamics. *PLoS One, 6*(10), e26379. doi: 10.1371/journal.pone.0026379.
49. George, S. P., Chen, H., Conrad, J. C., & Khurana, S. (2013). Regulation of directional cell migration by membrane-induced actin bundling. *Journal of Cell Science, 126*(2), 312–326. doi: 10.1242/jcs.117986.
50. Wakida, N. M., Botvinick, E. L., Lin, J., & Berns, M. W. (2010). An intact centrosome is required for the maintenance of polarization during directional cell migration. *PLoS One, 5*(12), e15462. doi: 10.1371/journal.pone.0015462.
51. Bre, M. H., Kreis, T. E., & Karsenti, E. (1987). Control of microtubule nucleation and stability in Madin-Darby canine kidney cells: The occurrence of noncentrosomal, stable detyrosinated microtubules. *Journal of Cell Biology, 105*(3), 1283–1296. doi: 10.1083/jcb.105.3.1283.
52. Hotani, H., & Horio, T. (1988). Dynamics of microtubules visualized by dark-field microscopy: Treadmilling and dynamic instability. *Cell Motility and the Cytoskeleton, 10*(3), 229–236. doi: 10.1002/cm.970100302.
53. Jordan, M. A., Toso, R. J., Thrower, D., & Wilson, L. (1993). Mechanism of mitotic block and inhibition of cell proliferation by taxol at low concentrations. *Proceedings of the National Academy of Sciences, 90*(20), 9552–9556. doi: 10.1073/pnas.90.20.9552.
54. Mitchison, T., & Kirschner, M. (1984). Dynamic instability of microtubule growth. *Nature, 312*(5991), 237–242. doi: 10.1038/312237a0.

55. Gundersen, G. G., & Bulinski, J. C. (1988). Selective stabilization of microtubules oriented toward the direction of cell migration. *Proceedings of the National Academy of Sciences, 85*(16), 5946–5950. doi: 10.1073/pnas.85.16.5946.
56. Bulinski, J. C., & Gundersen, G. G. (1991). Stabilization and post-translational modification of microtubules during cellular morphogenesis. *BioEssays, 13*(6), 285–294. doi: 10.1002/bies.950130607.
57. Webster, D. R., & Borisy, G. G. (1989). Microtubules are acetylated in domains that turn over slowly. *Journal of Cell Science, 92*(1), 57–65. doi: 10.1242/jcs.92.1.57.
58. Webster, D. R., Gundersen, G. G., Bulinski, J. C., & Borisy, G. G. (1987). Differential turnover of tyrosinated and detyrosinated microtubules. *Proceedings of the National Academy of Sciences, 84*(24), 9040–9044. doi: 10.1073/pnas.84.24.9040.
59. Webster, D. R., Gundersen, G. G., Bulinski, J. C., & Borisy, G. G. (1987). Assembly and turnover of detyrosinated tubulin in vivo. *Journal of Cell Biology, 105*(5), 265–276. doi: 10.1083/jcb.105.1.265.
60. Khawaja, S., Gundersen, G. G., & Bulinski, J. C. (1988). Enhanced stability of microtubules enriched in detyrosinated tubulin is not a direct function of detyrosination level. *Journal of Cell Biology, 106*(1), 141–149. doi: 10.1083/jcb.106.1.141.
61. Brady, S. T. (1995). A kinesin medley: Biochemical and functional heterogeneity. *Trends in Cell Biology, 5*(5), 159–164. doi: 10.1016/S0962-8924(00)88977-1.
62. Bhattacharya, A. B., Raha, B., & Bhattacharya, A. (2012). Losing the quantum state of microtubules to soul: Possibilities and challenges. *International Journal of Pharmaceutical Research and Bioscience, 1*, 315–328.
63. Bhattacharya, A. B., & Bhattacharya, A. (2015). Implementation of fuzzy technology in complicated medical diagnosis and further decision. In *Handbook of Research on Artificial Intelligence Techniques and Algorithms* (pp. 67–90). IGI Global. doi: 10.4018/978-1-4666-7240-6.ch004.

CHAPTER 3

The Inevitable Artificial Intelligence Revolution in Healthcare

SARTHAK GOEL, ANAMIKA GUHA, and B. K. TRIPATHY

School of Information Technology and Engineering,
Vellore Institute of Technology, Vellore, Tamil Nadu, India

ABSTRACT

The diagnosis of a disease is the first and the most important phase of a patient's treatment. Human errors can lead to miscalculated detection of disease, causing a delay in treatment, which can lead to irreversible damage like death. While physicians may diagnose the disease accurately, for a developing country like India where the doctor-to-citizen ratio is 1.34:1000, we need a cheap, accurate, scalable, and practical solution. Physicians rely on a cumbersome diagnosis process that can take months to diagnose. It is worth noting that diseases like Alzheimer's disease [2, 31] can have very long incubation periods and mild symptoms might make it difficult for not only the doctor to diagnose the disease but also the patient to report them. Dependence on Computed Tomography, Magnetic Resonance Imaging, fluorescent images, and continuous test reports can be tedious and expensive in rural areas, which makes us search for alternative technology.

The Internet of Things devices embedded in a fog computing architecture [4] can come to the rescue by bringing real-time processing and computing capability from a centralized server in a hospital right to the patient's bed [6]. Artificial Intelligence can rapidly analyze vast amounts of log data accumulated by clinically deployed Internet of Things devices

Data-Driven Analytics for Healthcare: Artificial Intelligence and Machine Learning for Medical Diagnostics.
Meghna Sharma, Priyanka Vashisht, A. V. Senthil Kumar, Chitra Singh, and Abdelmalek Amine (Eds.)

and identify the best treatment options. By using Artificial Intelligence in conjunction with medical judgment, these machines can promise new horizons in healthcare. In this chapter, let's explore the symbiosis of humans and machine intelligence, and discover how Artificial Intelligence is being put into action to diagnose fatal diseases and eliminate physician engagement. The chapter talks about how Deep Neural networks [32] can step into the boots of a physician to analyze data points like age, gender, smoking status, and blood pressure, and diagnose radiological, cardiovascular [3], dermatological, oncological disorders at a very early stage.

3.1 INTRODUCTION

As per a study conducted in 2014, published by the National Center for Biotechnology Information, out of 1,500 cases registered in the Amazon region, at least 600 would die of undiagnosed but treatable diseases. Human Immunodeficiency Virus-Associated Histoplasmosis is one of the highest contributing diseases in this region, causing more than 1,00,000 human immunodeficiency virus cases every year. Human immunodeficiency virus, which has an incubation period of about 3 months, comes with symptoms that are quite easily neglected during the early phases. Patients' negligence and the absence of proper healthcare facilities cause the virus to grow and continue to spread throughout the entire body. Only after there is a significant symptom, does the patient realize he is hosting a deadly disease in his body. Not just human immunodeficiency virus (HIV), hundreds of diseases like tumors, acquired immune deficiency syndrome, cardiovascular diseases [5] like coronary artery disease [21], and neurological diseases, can be fatal if not diagnosed at an early phase. Presently, much of the healthcare system is dependent on the physical workforce, which serves as a 1:1 model. Although very effective, this model lacks efficiency and scalability. With the increasing risks of chronic disease, there needs to be some mechanism that can cater to the treatment and diagnosis of a huge population. And thus, there arises a need for automating the entire healthcare system, by using the power of technology. Healthcare information systems have been adopted quite widely in private hospitals, which include portals to book appointments, store the medical history of the patient, make payments, search and book medical facilities, and inquire about information. Although these information systems eliminate paperwork to a huge extent, still human intervention is required at certain levels. Moreover, the user data collected by interactions with the portal can significantly facilitate hospitals in planning their infrastructure needs.

Machine Learning (ML) is a subset of Artificial Intelligence (AI) that feeds on data and can provide advanced techniques to diagnose diseases [7]. It is assisting doctors and physicians in identifying diseases by matching the symptoms with previous patients' data and thus predicting further steps. Computer Vision is being put to work with powerful Machine Learning algorithms to identify diseases pertaining to dermatology, radiology, oncology, and more. With high-performance Deep Learning (DL hereafter) algorithms that can analyze complex datasets of a patient's medical history, it's a matter of a few seconds to determine the cause and effect of any symptom. It is helping physicians to plan and take suitable actions. From analyzing drug interactions to drug discovery, Deep Neural Network-enabled simulations coupled with crystal clear graphics are facilitating physicians to detect and predict tumors, clotting disorders, and internal diseases that might have been hard to detect using traditional methods [34–36].

For a country like India, with a population of more than 1.4 billion people, Artificial Intelligence is likely to prove essential in solving the acute shortage of doctors. Moreover, it is a great solution for the Indian hospital industry, which is expected to increase at an annual growth rate of 16–17%, as mentioned by the India Brand Equity Foundation (IBEF) [25]. Scientists are turning large amounts of medical data into actionable facts that are being fed into highly efficient algorithms to produce targeted research and development and accelerate health responses [10, 33]. Artificial Intelligence is assisting physicians by providing a complete picture of all the possible different diagnosis combinations, from which doctors can derive the right conclusions. Data is facilitating scientists to predict which sector of the population is likely to face health issues soon by analyzing their eating patterns.

3.2 ARTIFICIAL INTELLIGENCE (AI)

In this section, we provide a brief overview of Artificial Intelligence, and how it works, and aim to showcase its capabilities. Artificial Intelligence, in simple terms, involves giving machines the ability to think or be intelligent. The goal is to make machines smart enough to perform repetitive tasks with minimal variations. While the term "artificial intelligence" was coined in 1956 [19], subsets of AI have been in use for a long time. One popular way to classify AI is into three categories:

3.2.1 GENERAL PURPOSE ARTIFICIAL INTELLIGENCE (DEEP ARTIFICIAL INTELLIGENCE/STRONG ARTIFICIAL INTELLIGENCE)

This refers to the ability of an intelligent agent to imitate human intelligence. It typically involves a combination of specialized AI machines to create a system that can think, understand, learn, and apply concepts to solve real-world problems. Examples include self-driving cars and advanced robots. Strong artificial intelligence possesses processing capabilities similar to humans, using common sense, background knowledge, abstraction, and transfer learning enforced through reinforcement learning with deep neural networks to mimic human-like problem-solving. While rare, such strong AI systems can solve complex problems, but they can be very expensive and time-consuming. For instance, the supercomputer Kei by Fujitsu took around 40 minutes to simulate a single second of neural activity, highlighting the resource-intensive nature of strong artificial intelligence systems.

3.2.2 ARTIFICIAL SUPER INTELLIGENCE

Self-explanatory by its name, this classification of artificial intelligence describes a machine more intelligent than humans. It is on par with concepts understood by mankind and is expected to provide a better understanding of complex systems like the human body, the universe, and atomic interactions. This type of artificial intelligence is expected to solve several mysteries of nature; however, as one would anticipate, achieving Artificial superintelligence is preserved in the womb of the future. The closest examples we can relate to are from science fiction movies.

3.2.3 SPECIAL PURPOSE ARTIFICIAL INTELLIGENCE (NARROW ARTIFICIAL INTELLIGENCE)

Chatbots, recommendation engines, predicting systems, natural language processing systems, and computer vision systems, all constitute narrow artificial intelligence as they specialize in one area. It is one of the most widely researched fields of artificial intelligence with more than 1,00,000 papers published, concerning different applications. Most healthcare applications find their way into this category only.

3.2.3.1 MACHINE LEARNING

1. **Supervised Learning:** The algorithms in this category use labeled datasets that are used to predict or classify target attributes [19]. Logistic regression, Support Vector Models, and Neural Networks [38], generally fall under this category.

2. **Unsupervised Learning:** Generally, these types of algorithms are used to reveal hidden patterns in unlabeled datasets, usually by statistical methods. Cluster Analysis is one of the widely used algorithms under this category. These algorithms have the power to identify relationships between data values.

3. **Reinforcement Learning:** A reward-based application of machine learning algorithms, where the agent is trained with negative and positive reinforcement to improve the accuracy of the model. It usually finds its way into gaming and robotic applications.

3.2.3.2 DEEP LEARNING (DL)

A subset of machine learning enables computers to filter features, which could be in the form of text or multimedia, to classify and/or predict the target variable. Inspired by the way the human brain functions, it attempts to mimic the way neurons process information. For complex applications involving multimedia such as images and audio [37, 39], traditional machine learning doesn't yield the best results as they specialize in text and numeric data. The layered architecture of deep learning algorithms allows it to decide which parameters are suitable for a given use case. This feature of deep learning is highly useful when there is little domain knowledge about the dataset. Just like machine learning, there exist several deep learning techniques, such as Convolutional Neural Networks [37], Recurrent Neural Networks, and so on. Each of these specializes in some use case. These nonlinear processing units form the layered architecture used for feature extraction and transformation. Each layer uses output from the previous layer and tries to learn from a hierarchy of concepts. Based on the findings, the weights are adjusted based on the network propagation direction. For example, in the case of processing an image, the first layer might convert the image into a matrix of pixels and encode it. The next layer would use this matrix to remove noise from the image and encode the edges. The consecutive layer now has a matrix that is free from noise and can encode eyes and lips. Finally, the final layer recognizes that the image is essentially of a face. With weight adjustments and tuning, the algorithm improves its efficiency to deliver better results. This iterative yet powerful approach makes deep learning extremely useful in the healthcare domain. Unlike traditional image transformation algorithms, Deep Learning (DL) is more data-intensive and efficient. With medical images readily available, deep learning algorithms can deliver significantly accurate results through object recognition.

3.3 LITERATURE REVIEW AND BACKGROUND

To better understand how artificial intelligence can use enormous medical data available to deliver insights and diagnose a patient's disease, we first review related studies on the topic. These include surveys about the progress artificial intelligence has made in healthcare [7, 11, 13], the evolution of algorithms, how robotics [19, 27], the Internet of Things, computer vision, and natural language processing are coming into action to facilitate deep learning algorithms for expanding the adoption of this powerful technology [14]. We also review the trust between humans and the findings of Artificial Intelligence Algorithms [9]. Knowledge embodiment is a related field that uses social informatics perspectives that aim at developing Artificial Intelligence-based robotics systems [27]. It provides arguments that support the embodiment of Artificial Intelligence technologies with human knowledge and capabilities and thus paves the way for further social informatics studies of Artificial Intelligence technologies in disease diagnostics, making it a more active and autonomous social actor. Knowledge embodiment in Artificial Intelligence systems is useful in creating smart assistants [15] that can understand a patient's symptoms in natural language and abstract all the processing to output feedback in layman's grammar.

Ashish [7] in his article mentions how Artificial Intelligence is evolving the existing diagnosis methods by digitizing the traditional methods. The contribution of Artificial Intelligence in the diagnosis of Dermatology, Radiology, and Drug Design are the focus areas of this chapter.

Artificial Intelligence finds its way into treatment design and diagnosis, drug designing and simulating environments to test its efficiency, skin cancer recognition, and classification, MRI scans, and assisted surgery. Another source sheds light on different artificial intelligence techniques in healthcare [11], where leading techniques include support vector machines, extreme learning machines, the internet of things, convolutional neural networks, and Mobile Agents. In Ref. [8], we explore some current and future use cases of Artificial Intelligence in healthcare, which include precision diagnostics, precision therapeutics, precision medicine, virtual assistants, and Artificial Intelligence chatbots, immunomes and synthetic biology, and Artificial Intelligence-driven drug discovery. Furthermore, we reviewed some disease-specific articles that provided an understanding of how artificial intelligence-based algorithms are aiding in diagnosing complex neurological and cardiovascular disorders. The authors touch upon different disorders like Alzheimer's disease, Parkinson's disease [18], breast cancer, lung cancer, and cardiovascular diseases. Comparisons of different possible algorithms were referred to, which provided a deeper understanding of possible solutions artificial intelligence can bring to this sector. Trust issues between humans and results generated by artificial intelligence algorithms were also referred to in Refs. [9, 13] to analyze if people are ready to accept recommendations and predictions made by artificial intelligence assistants. An interesting study [17] discussed how artificial intelligence-based advanced algorithms are assisting in drug development for cancer. Deep learning-based algorithms are generating possible results for every drug interaction by simulating the human body. This is further being analyzed to create a sustainable drug delivery mechanism by the use of Transfer Learning [28]. Finally, we also review the impact of cloud computing, the internet of Things, and edge computing in healthcare [29]. Fog computing reduces the network latency, bandwidth bottleneck, and transmission delays involved in the traditional cloud-based processing framework [30]. Using distributed computing and a k-fold random forest algorithm, this approach achieves a 92% accuracy and reduces the latency by approximately 95% compared to existing traditional models. Internet of Things-enabled sensors like body sensors are being used to send raw data to storage servers on the cloud, which use deep learning-enabled algorithms to extract features and provide insights. Decision support systems then compare the findings with rules from the database. All of this is creating a self-support ecosystem for the patient, making it less dependent on doctors. Artificial Intelligence is making a breakthrough in biomedical applications by answering questions using the Natural Language Processing technique referred to as the Biomedical Question Answering Framework (BioQA) [23]. Text classification algorithms reduce the question to a basic yes-or-no answer-based statement.

3.4 DISCUSSION

With the accumulation of this huge data, artificial intelligence can be used to deliver significant insights. This chapter explores how data collected via healthcare devices can be put into action to not only predict but also diagnose diseases and disorders in humans. No doubt, smart machines can never replace physicians; however, both can work complementary to each other, giving benefits to the end user, i.e., the patient. The most basic way artificial intelligence can contribute to the healthcare sector is by analyzing the past medical history of a patient and applying a couple of algorithms to predict or diagnose if he is suffering from a particular disease. It can be a classification or regression use case where the algorithm delivers a Yes or No output or determines the probability of him suffering from the disease, helping physicians to narrow down possible diseases a patient has. This technique is being widely used today and is even being deployed in some mobile applications, which makes the patient self-sufficient to get a blunt idea of what he is suffering from. Seeing the rise in cardiovascular disease, several Mobile Health (mHealth) technologies have made their way to the market. Mobile health applications provide physical activity trackers, dietary monitoring apps, and blood pressure monitors that can suggest preventive habits to achieve target levels. Apple Heart Study application is one such application that is essentially a pulse rate data analyzer [19]. Healthcare Internet of Things devices such as connected inhalers, Internet of Things-based connected inhalers, ingestible sensors, and more are being used as data-producing agents, while Fog computing is helping in bringing high computing power right to the patient's monitoring system. Gene Expression is an interesting diagnostic tool that classifies and detects abnormalities by interpreting microarray data using machine learning-based algorithms [23].

Today, high computing power is available at our fingertips, at a little expense. Achieving powerful simulations to imitate the action of a drug on a human can save the lives of test subjects. Deep learning algorithms

[1] specialize in imitating the characteristics of a human or animal who is the target of a drug, still in the research phase. Developing simulations can explore a lot of possible opportunities such as experimenting with the drug, trying different permutations and combinations with drugs, attempting diagnosis in different fashions, and thereby reducing the cost of tests significantly, with no threat of aftereffects. Analytical tools, when integrated with machine learning algorithms, render interesting visualizations that reveal discoveries. These can help organizations make far-sighted decisions and collaborate with patients at an early stage. Powerful Artificial Neural Network-based object detection algorithms are handling the repetitive tasks of analyzing X-rays, Computed Tomography Scans, test reports, and delivering insights from timestamped medical data as precise as 1 millisecond. Artificial Intelligence Algorithms have reduced the time to diagnose diseases from weeks to hours. Whether it's a common cold, flu, or cancer, deep learning algorithms are improving in diagnosing them.

Artificial Intelligence now covers a wide range of applications such as signal and image processing to predict changes in the functioning of body organs like urinary bladder control, stroke predictions, and tropical diseases [23]. More importantly, it is being utilized as a Decision Support System (DSS).

3.4.1 ARTIFICIAL INTELLIGENCE IN DIAGNOSING SKIN CANCER

It is expected that more than 6.3 billion people use deep learning-enabled mobile subscription services to detect skin cancers [24]. Using the HAM1000 dataset, researchers utilized 80% of images to feed them to convolutional neural network-based models – DenseNet 201, ResNet152, Inception_V4 to achieve a confusion matrix of 0.96, 0.96, 0.96 [7]. Transfer learning is another possible technology that can diagnose skin cancer. AlexNet is one such algorithm.

3.4.2 ARTIFICIAL INTELLIGENCE TO DIAGNOSE CARDIOVASCULAR DISEASE (CVD)

Artificial intelligence techniques have gained a lot of popularity in diagnosing cardiovascular diseases. While 85 million people were affected in one way or another by cardiovascular disease, the figure keeps on growing [19]. This costs more than 210 billion euros in Europe alone, accounting for around 53% of all healthcare costs. Deep Learning and cognitive computing have the potential to revolutionize the way we look at cardiovascular diseases. Even electronic health records are sources of information, useful in training algorithms to predict diseases [12, 22]. They provide several useful features like age, ancestry, ethnicity, insurance, gender, and many more that can be used to train models and derive interesting results.

3.4.3 ECHO CARDIOGRAPHY

A very crucial step in diagnosing and managing cardiovascular diseases is assessing the cardiac structure and functioning of the heart. In traditional systems, it depends on the experience of the doctor to diagnose any cardiovascular disease by manually analyzing test results. ML models, however, can enable even non-expert clinicians to do the job. By training models with a wide variety of medical images containing specific disease patterns, analyzing the relationship of each pixel, artificial intelligence can automate the job of cardiovascular diagnosis. Artificial Intelligence opens up tons of interesting opportunities such as 3D echocardiography that gives interactive outputs, enabling even a layman to understand the concepts of volume of atrium and ventricle, systolic/diastolic flow, ejection fraction from ventricles. These customizable algorithms can animate medical images to simulate the functioning of patients' hearts in real-time, which enables doctors to experiment with the simulation and find the best suitable practice. Cognitive machine learning is applied here while scientists train machine learning algorithms with echocardiographic data to understand restrictive cardiomyopathy and constrictive pericarditis. Even simple supervised and unsupervised learning algorithms provide ample opportunities such as analyzing the functioning of the heart valve or aortic valve, while complex deep learning-based models can use a combination of neural networks and merge the outcome to find even more accurate results such as disease severity score, survival prediction factor, etc. [20].

3.4.4 MAGNETIC RESONANCE IMAGING [18]

Popularly known as MRI, convolutional neural networks and stacked autoencoders trained using a magnetic resonance imaging specific dataset are being widely used for automatic detection and segmentation of heart ventricles.

3.4.5 CARDIAC COMPUTED TOMOGRAPHY

Image analysis is being extensively used in cardiac computed tomography for diagnosing coronary artery disease (CAD) and atherosclerosis. Machine Learning algorithms replace the traditional practices of analyzing coronary computed tomographic angiography tests. Machine Learning models are providing clinical value by characterizing coronary plaque and coronary artery calcium scoring thereby reducing false positives. Using texture analysis, machine learning algorithms can now detect prognosis and myocardial infarctions.

3.4.6 ELECTROCARDIOGRAPHY

Electrocardiography (ECG) is the most widely and commonly used method of diagnosing any cardiovascular disease. Deep Learning algorithms can automatically detect anomalies from electrocardiography scripts, thereby signaling disease. Deep Neural Networks are being used for electrocardiography interpretation optimization, arrhythmia classification, and systolic dysfunction detection which is outperforming the existing brain natriuretic peptide blood test screening process.

3.5 ARTIFICIAL INTELLIGENCE IN MAGNETIC RESONANCE IMAGING CLASSIFICATION TASK OF HUMAN BRAIN NEUROLOGICAL [18]

A non-invasive and painless medical imaging technique that is widely adopted across the world, is fundamental for detection, diagnosis, and treatment of the disease. Functional Magnetic Resonance Imaging yields high spatial resolution images that are suitable for training deep learning models that achieve more efficient and improved results. Out of the available algorithms, Support Vector Machine-based algorithms have been widely used. With more than 2,000 publications on support vector machines, it outperforms artificial neural networks, random forest, logistic regression, K-nearest neighbor, and Naive Bayes. Though algorithms like AdaBoost and gradient boost algorithms might be more accurate, researchers are finding it difficult to relate with medical use cases. Support vector machine promises most accurate and efficient results with less false positives. 2D and 3D Convolutional Neural Networks are also suitable alternatives for Support Vector Machine; though they too take high compute power and time to build the model. Some important applications in human brain, where artificial intelligence can perform image processing tasks are as in subsections.

3.5.1 ALZHEIMER'S DISEASE

A neurodegenerative disorder that accounts for more than 60% of dementia. It is a symptom of loss of short-term memory which results in language disorder, emotional instability, disorientation, and several behavioral problems. With artificial intelligence, scientists have achieved remarkable results by analyzing magnetic resonance images. Naive Bayes, artificial neural networks, k-Nearest Neighbor, support vector machine [11] are among the top-performing models in this category. With a combined accuracy of 98%, these classifiers outperform any physician. The 3D-Convolutional neural network models with visual inspection tools including sensitivity analysis, 3D mapping, though yield a limited accuracy of about 80%, still deliver a lot of insights about the medical image dataset. Combining other algorithms like Long Short-Term Memory (LSTM), Convolutional Neural Network (CNN), Generative Adversarial Network (GAN), and Transfer Learning with basic classifiers can provide accurate results.

3.5.2 PARKINSON'S DISEASE

A chronic neurodegenerative disorder which affects the nervous system of a patient causing tremor, limb stiffness, emotional problems, sleep, and decreased motor function. Generative Neural Networks, 3D-Convolutional Neural Networks, K-Nearest Neighbor, Support Vector Machine, Random Forest, Naïve Bayes, Transfer learning are some of the possible algorithms contributing towards diagnosing Parkinson's Disease (PD). 3D-Convolutional Neural Networks have been able to achieve accuracy as high as 100%, while Support Vector Machine, K-Nearest Neighbor, and Naïve Bayes deliver a 99% accuracy for men and 96.9% accuracy for women. Autism Spectrum Disorder, Major Depressive Disorder, Schizophrenia are some other use cases where deep learning algorithms like support vector machines and 3D–4D Convolutional Neural Networks models are making an impact by providing powerful analytical capabilities.

3.6 ARTIFICIAL INTELLIGENCE IN MAMMOGRAPHIC PHENOTYPING OF BREAST CANCER [16]

Artificial Intelligence has delivered ambitious results by generalizing its findings across diverse datasets, with different architectures. Reproducibility, generalizability, and interpretability are the three key factors during the assessment. Currently, full-field digital mammography is the leading dataset for breast cancer detection, which includes imaging from years even prior to artificial intelligence's adoption in cancer diagnosis. Artificial Neural Networks, Bayesian Networks, Support Vector Machines, and decision trees are widely used algorithms for this use case. Generally, all the aforementioned algorithms yield comparable results. Support Vector Machines generally outperform other classifiers in terms of accuracy; however, it takes more time to build the model. A comparative graph between different classifiers is shown in Figure 3.1.

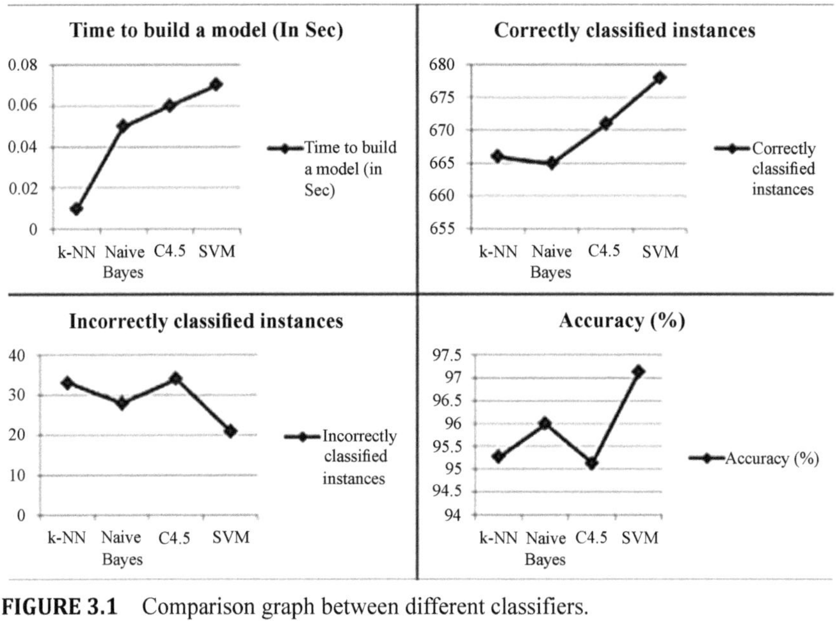

FIGURE 3.1 Comparison graph between different classifiers.

3.7 ARTIFICIAL INTELLIGENCE A FRAMEWORK TO PREDICT LUNG CANCER PROGNOSIS [26]

Lung cancer took more than 1,50,000 lives in 2018 in the United States alone, which accounts for around 25% of all cancer deaths (American Cancer Society). The National Cancer Institute of the United States estimates an increase of 30% in new cases and mortality rate of lung cancer in this decade. Artificial Intelligence can help predict lung cancer patients' as well as increase their survival chances by analyzing their day-to-day activities and exposure to carcinogens. Contrary to traditional statistical methods used by doctors and physicians, artificial intelligence proposes advanced algorithms that can model the non-linear relationships without imposing assumptions. With a diverse choice of dataset, artificial intelligence algorithms can work on genetic data, pathological images, tumor characteristics, and other complex datasets. Support Vector Machines and Deep Learning based Bayesian network models estimate survival rates even with sparse and inconsistent dataset. Applied multiple decision trees efficiently classify lung cancer cases, based on gene expression levels to estimate cancer survival prediction. From simple algorithms like Logistic Regression and Decision Tree-based models to complex Artificial Neural Network-based algorithms, all contribute in some way or another. Today, Artificial Neural Networks-based methods are providing a robust approach for regression and classification problems. Algorithms are implicitly learning from complex, noisy data which includes X-ray images, medical records, etc. Naive Bayes classifiers and K-Fold cross-validation models are more algorithms contributing to artificial intelligence in healthcare use cases.

3.8 ARTIFICIAL INTELLIGENCE TO DIAGNOSE RETINAL DISEASE

This involves the use of two stages, where the first one is creating deep segmented images and diagnosing the patient, the second one being a double-layered Convolutional Neural Network that uses segmented images to diagnose disorders [7]. Diabetic Retinopathy is extensively used today, especially after it received the United States Food and Drug Administration's approval in 2018. It involves uploading a retina image of the patient to the algorithm, which classifies retinal condition as high, mild, and low diabetic retinopathy [40]. Additionally, personalized treatments and precautions are also generated for the patient in real time. The Inner

Eye deep learning toolkit provides a quantitative radiology mechanism suitable for monitoring tumor progression, which is essential for planning surgery and radiotherapy [8].

3.9 CHALLENGES

Even though artificial intelligence promises a better and more capable healthcare industry, there are a lot of challenges that arise, especially in the early phase. The promise of artificial intelligence and the opportunities it will bring in the healthcare sector are evident in this chapter. Seeing the increasing demand for skilled doctors, Computer-Aided Diagnosis (CAD) is the future. Fast, accurate, consistent, and reliable are some of the traits of computer-aided design (CAD) results. However, there are some equally important challenges.

3.9.1 DATA ARTIFICIAL INTELLIGENCE LIABILITY

Artificial Intelligence relies on data. Clean and consistent data promises relevant results. At the same time, the availability of huge datasets guarantees more acceptable results. However, often, even a small manipulation in data can significantly impact the results. For healthcare applications, where every life is precious, experimenting on live patients can be lethal. The solution to this challenge is the availability of verified and cleaned data that can be readily used for processing.

3.9.2 DATA MANAGEMENT

Medical data can contain personal information that can reveal the personal identity of the patient [7, 13]. Though this information might be useful for pharmaceutical and healthcare industries, from a security point of view, not many patients are comfortable sharing their identity. Hence, there needs to be some standards and regulations to bind organizations from sharing data.

3.9.3 ALGORITHMIC COMPLEXITY AND ARCHITECTURE

While cloud computing might guarantee high processing power, the algorithm and architecture of an algorithm still play a big role in decreasing the time complexity. Inefficient architectures mean long computing times, which may not be feasible for the organization. Consulting a physician is a wiser choice than waiting for hours to diagnose a common cold using advanced algorithms and petabytes of data. Hence, algorithms need to be optimized and specific to use cases.

During the early training phases, artificial intelligence is bound to make mistakes. Giving wrong recommendations, making inaccurate predictions, or diagnosing the wrong disease is a possibility during the initial years of research. Acceptable in some sectors, these mistakes can lead to further wrong actions that can cost a patient their life. The availability of technical infrastructure, especially in rural areas, is another major challenge [8].

3.10 CONCLUSION

Artificial Intelligence is indeed one of the most significant inventions ever made by humans. With quintillion bytes of data being produced every day, artificial intelligence is one of the few technologies that can process it to provide value to businesses. Moreover, using artificial intelligence's sister technologies like Internet of Things, Computer Vision, Robotics, and Automation can be used to invent revolutionary products. Intelligent robots that can replace nurses and supporting staff will eventually become a reality in the near future. Developed countries have started replacing chemists with automated vending machines, which use computer vision algorithms to read prescriptions and dispense required medicines using a robotic arm, while the payment is done digitally. Powerful deep learning algorithms are helping doctors identify blockages, tumors, and signs of possible diseases in patients' medical data. Regression algorithms make it easy for doctors to predict the chances of encountering a particular disease by analyzing eating habits, blood pressure levels, oxygen levels, and glucose levels, which are automatically collected by Internet of Things devices. All these advancements indicate that the onset of artificial intelligence is going to change, once and for all, the way the healthcare industry works. Doctors can focus on finding creative ways to cure diseases, while artificially intelligent assistants would diagnose diseases and provide personalized remedies to patients.

KEYWORDS

- **artificial intelligence**
- **deep learning**
- **fog computing**
- **healthcare**
- **internet of things**
- **regression algorithms**

REFERENCES

1. Kavitha, M., Jayasankar, T., Venkatesh, P., Mani, G., Bharatiraja, C., & Twala, B. (2021). COVID-19 disease diagnosis using smart DL techniques. *Journal of Applied Science and Engineering, 24*(3), 271–277. Retrieved from: http://jase.tku.edu.tw/articles/jase-202106-24-3-0001 (accessed on 31 May 2024).
2. Mirbabaie, M., Stieglitz, S., & Frick, N. (2021). AI in disease diagnostics: A critical review and classification on the current state of research guiding future direction. *Health and Technology, 11*(4), 693–731. doi: 10.1007/s12553-021-00555-5.
3. Ghosh, P., et al. (2021). Efficient prediction of cardiovascular disease using ML algorithms with Relief and LASSO feature selection techniques. *IEEE Access, 9*, 19304–19326. doi: 10.1109/ACCESS.2021.3053759.
4. Awaisi, K. S., Hussain, S., Ahmed, M., Khan, A. A., & Ahmed, G. (2020). Leveraging IoT and fog computing in healthcare systems. *IEEE Internet of Things Magazine, 3*(2), 52–56. doi: 10.1109/IOTM.0001.1900096.
5. Swathy, M., & Saruladha, K. (2022). A comparative study of classification and prediction of cardiovascular diseases (CVD) using ML and DL techniques. *ICT Express, 8*(1), 109–116. Available from: https://www.sciencedirect.com/science/article/pii/S2405959521001119 (accessed on 31 May 2024).
6. Pareek, K., Tiwari, P. K., & Bhatnagar, V. (2021). Fog computing in healthcare: A review. *IOP Conference Series: Materials Science and Engineering, 1099*(1), 012025. doi: 10.1088/1757-899x/1099/1/012025.
7. Manne, R., & Kantheti, S. (2021). Application of AI in healthcare: Chances and challenges. *Current Journal of Applied Science and Technology, 40*, 78–89. doi: 10.9734/CJAST/2021/v40i631320.
8. Bajwa, J., Munir, U., Nori, A., & Williams, B. (2021). AI in healthcare: Transforming the practice of medicine. *Future Healthcare Journal, 8*(2), e188–e194. doi: 10.7861/fhj.2021-0095.

9. Asan, O., Bayrak, A., & Choudhury, A. (2020). AI and human trust in healthcare: Focus on clinicians. *Journal of Medical Internet Research, 22*(6), e15154. doi: 10.2196/15154.
10. Bajpai, N., & Wadhwa, M. (2021). Artificial intelligence and healthcare in India (pp. 7, 10). *ICT India Working Papers, 43*. Center for Sustainable Development, Earth Institute, Columbia University. https://doi.org/10.7916/d8-v30w-7139.
11. Gaikwad, S. (2021). Study on AI in healthcare. *7th International Conference on Advanced Computing and Communication Systems (ICACCS), 2021*, 1165–1169. doi: 10.1109/ICACCS51430.2021.9441741.
12. Parashar, G., Chaudhary, A., & Rana, A. (2021). Systematic mapping study of AI/ML in healthcare and future directions. *SN Computer Science, 2*(6), 461. doi: 10.1007/s42979-021-00848-6.
13. Gómez-González, E., Gomez, E., Márquez-Rivas, J., Guerrero-Claro, M., Fernández-Lizaranzu, I., Relimpio-López, M. I., Dorado, M. E., Mayorga-Buiza, M. J., Izquierdo-Ayuso, G., & Capitán-Morales, L. (2020). Artificial intelligence in medicine and healthcare: A review and classification of current and near-future applications and their ethical and social impact. arXiv. https://arxiv.org/abs/2001.09778.
14. Apell, P., & Eriksson, H. (2023). Artificial intelligence (AI) healthcare technology innovations: the current state and challenges from a life science industry perspective. *Technology Analysis & Strategic Management, 35*(2), 179–193. DOI: 10.1080/09537325.2021.1971188.
15. Health, V. S., Drysdale, E., Dolatabadi, E., Chivers, C., Liu, V., Saria, S., Sendak, M., Wiens, J., Brudno, M., Hoyt, A., Mazwi, M., Mamdani, M., Singh, Allen, V., McGregor, C., Ross, H., Szeto, A., Anand, A., Verma, & Wang, B. (2019). Implementing AI in healthcare. Vector Institute, 4, 6, 17. Retrieved from https://vectorinstitute.ai/wp-content/uploads/2020/03/implementing-ai-in-healthcare.pdf.
16. Gastounioti, A., Desai, S., Ahluwalia, V. S., et al. (2022). AI in mammographic phenotyping of breast cancer risk: A narrative review. *Breast Cancer Research, 24*, 14. doi: 10.1186/s13058-022-01509-z.
17. Liang, G., Fan, W., Luo, H., & Zhu, H. (2020). The emerging roles of AI in cancer drug development and precision therapy. *Biomedicine & Pharmacotherapy, 128*, 110255. doi: 10.1016/j.biopha.2020.110255.
18. Zhang, Z., Li, G., Xu, Y., & Tang, X. (2021). Application of AI in the MRI classification task of human brain neurological and psychiatric diseases: A scoping review. *Diagnostics, 11*(8), 1402. doi: 10.3390/diagnostics11081402.
19. Romiti, S., Vinciguerra, M., Saade, W., Cortajarena, I. A., & Greco, E. (2020). AI and cardiovascular diseases: An unexpected alliance. *Cardiology Research and Practice, 2020*, 4972346. doi: 10.1155/2020/4972346.
20. Chang, V., Bhavani, V., Xu, A., & Hossain, M. (2022). An AI model for heart disease detection using ML algorithms. *Healthcare Analytics, 2*, 100016. doi: 10.1016/j.health.2022.100016.
21. Gautam, N., Saluja, P., Malkawi, A., Rabbat, M. G., Al-Mallah, M. H., Pontone, G., Zhang, Y., Lee, B. C., & Al'Aref, S. J. (2022). Current and future applications of AI in coronary artery disease. *Healthcare (Basel, Switzerland), 10*(2), 232. https://doi.org/10.3390/healthcare10020232.

22. Wesołowski, S., Lemmon, G., Hernandez, E. J., Henrie, A., Miller, T. A., Weyhrauch, D., et al. (2022). An explainable AI approach for predicting cardiovascular outcomes using electronic health records. *PLOS Digital Health, 1*(1), e0000004. https://doi.org/10.1371/journal.pdig.0000004.
23. Rong, G., Mendez, A., BouAssi, E., Zhao, B., & Sawan, M. (2020). AI in healthcare: Review and prediction case studies. *Engineering, 6*(3), 291–301. doi: 10.1016/j.eng.2019.08.015.
24. Shelmerdine, S. C., Arthurs, O. J., Denniston, A., & Sebire, N. J. (2021). Review of study reporting guidelines for clinical studies using AI in healthcare. *BMJ Health & Care Informatics, 28*(1), e100385. https://doi.org/10.1136/bmjhci-2021-100385.
25. Prema, R. K., Kathiravan, M., & Shaikh, A. A. (2021). AI in healthcare: 21st century age of rifles – A bibliometric analysis. *Asia Pacific Journal of Health Management, 16*(4), 274–281. https://doi.org/10.24083/apjhm.v16i4.1327.
26. Johnson, M., Albizri, A., & Simsek, S. (2022). AI in healthcare operations to enhance treatment outcomes: A framework to predict lung cancer prognosis. *Annals of Operations Research, 308*, 275–305. https://doi.org/10.1007/s10479-020-03872-6.
27. Pee, L. G., Pan, S. L., & Cui, L. (2018). AI in healthcare robots: A social informatics study of knowledge embodiment. *Journal of the Association for Information Science and Technology, 70*(4), 351–369. https://doi.org/10.1002/asi.24145.
28. Manish, K. M. (2021). AI in healthcare. *International Journal of Advanced Research in Science, Communication and Technology (IJARSCT), 10*(1), 147–148. https://doi.org/10.48175/568.
29. Ijaz, M., Li, G., Lin, L., Cheikhrouhou, O., Hamam, H., & Noor, M. (2021). Integration and applications of fog computing and cloud computing based on the internet of things for provision of healthcare services at home. *Electronics, 10*, 1077. https://doi.org/10.3390/electronics10091077.
30. Kishor, A., Chakraborty, C., & Jeberson, W. (2021). A novel fog computing approach for minimization of latency in healthcare using ML. *International Journal of Interactive Multimedia & AI, 6*(7), 7–17. https://doi.org/10.9781/ijimai.2020.12.004.
31. Singhania, U., Tripathy, B., Hasan, M. K., Ahmed, T. E., & Nour, M. M. M. (2021). A predictive and preventive model for onset of Alzheimer's disease. *Frontiers in Public Health, 9*, 751536.
32. Bhattacharyya, S., Snasel, V., Hassanian, A. E., Saha, S., & Tripathy, B. K. (2020). Chapter 3 in *Deep Learning Research with Engineering Applications* (Vol. 7, 1st ed., pp. 51). De Gruyter Publications. doi: 10.1515/9783110670905.
33. Kaul, D., Raju, H., & Tripathy, B. K. (2022). DL in healthcare. In Acharjya, D. P., Mitra, A., Zaman, N. (Eds.), *DL in Data Analytics – Recent Techniques, Practices and Applications* (pp. 97–115). Studies in Big Data, vol. 91. Springer, Cham. doi: 10.1007/978-3-030-75855-4_6.
34. Tripathy, B. K., & Adate, A. (2021). Impact of deep neural learning on AI research. In D. P. Acharjya, A. Mitra, & N. Zaman (Eds.), *DL in Data Analytics – Recent Techniques, Practices and Applications* (pp. 145–170). Studies in Big Data, vol. 91. Springer, Cham. doi: 10.1007/978-3-030-75855-4_9.
35. Adate, A., & Tripathy, B. K. (2020). Impact of deep neural learning on AI research. In S. Bhattacharyya, A. E. Hassanian, S. Saha, & B. K. Tripathy (Eds.), *DL Research and Applications* (pp. 69–84). De Gruyter Publications. doi: 10.1515/9783110670905-004.

36. Maheswari, K., Shaha, A., Arya, D., Tripathy, B. K., & Rajkumar, R. (2020). Convolutional neural networks: A bottom-up approach. In S. Bhattacharyya, A. E. Hassanian, S. Saha, & B. K. Tripathy (Eds.), *DL Research with Engineering Applications* (pp. 21–50). De Gruyter Publications. doi: 10.1515/9783110670905-002.
37. Tripathy, B. K., Parikh, S., Ajay, P., & Magapu, C. (2022). Brain MRI segmentation techniques based on CNN and its variants. In J. Chaki (Ed.), *Brain Tumor MRI Image Segmentation Using DL Techniques* (pp. 161–182). Elsevier Publications. doi: 10.1016/B978-0-323-91171-9.000.
38. Tripathy, B. K., & Anuradha, J. (2018). *Soft Computing: Advances and Applications* (1st ed., pp. 325–329). Cengage India. ISBN 978–8131526194.
39. Bose, A., & Tripathy, B. K. (2020). DL for audio signal classification. In S. Bhattacharyya, A. E. Hassanian, S. Saha, & B. K. Tripathy (Eds.), *DL Research and Applications* (pp. 105–136). De Gruyter Publications. https://doi.org/10.1515/9783110670905-00660.
40. Prabhavathy, P., Tripathy, B. K., & Venkatesan, M. (2022). Analysis of diabetic retinopathy detection techniques using CNN models. In S. Mishra, H. K. Tripathy, P. Mallick, & K. Shaalan (Eds.), *Augmented Intelligence in Healthcare: A Pragmatic and Integrated Analysis* (Studies in Computational Intelligence, vol 1024, pp. 161–182). Springer, Singapore. https://doi.org/10.1007/978-981-19-1076-0_6.

CHAPTER 4

Object Detection Approach for Pneumonia Detection Using X-Ray Images

TANISHQ VARSHNEY and RUCHI SEHRAWAT

Department of Computer Science, University School of Information, Communication, and Technology, GGSIPU, Delhi, India

ABSTRACT

Pneumonia is an infectious disease; people may face this disease at any period of their lives. Prevalent symptoms like fever and cold are often seen in patients. There are various methods like CT-scan, MRI, and chest radiographs available for diagnosing this disease. X-ray images are the most common, reliable, and efficient way of detecting pneumonia in human lungs. RSNA Pneumonia detection is the dataset used for this research study. This dataset contains three classes: lung opacity class with 6,012 instances, abnormal class with 11,821 images, and normal class with 8,851 images. These X-ray images are used to train the model. The object detection model is first trained on the given dataset and then will be able to classify and detect the position of pneumonia in human lungs. There are various machine learning and deep learning approaches available, but most of them are just classifying the images based on whether that disease exists or not. Healthcare is considered one of the important sectors. There is a continuous need for automated systems to make them reliable. This study emphasizes on providing a reliable and efficient deep learning approach for detecting pneumonia in the lungs. A mask R-CNN model which helps in detecting and localizing the lung opacity is built.

Data-Driven Analytics for Healthcare: Artificial Intelligence and Machine Learning for Medical Diagnostics. Meghna Sharma, Priyanka Vashisht, A. V. Senthil Kumar, Chitra Singh, and Abdelmalek Amine (Eds.)

This model uses ResNet-50 architecture as its backbone. Bounding boxes are used to locate the disease by detecting lung opacities in X-ray images. This model shows desirable results. This model can be deployed in real-time scenarios to detect pneumonia. This makes the process of detecting pneumonia in human lungs a lot cheaper and quicker.

4.1 INTRODUCTION

Pneumonia is one of the infectious seasonal diseases that occur in human lungs and can range in severity from mild to a major life-threatening problem for children (age <5) and senior citizens (age >60) [1]. Pneumonia symptoms range from moderate to severe, depending on the type of germ that caused the illness. Mild signs and symptoms are sometimes mistaken for those of a cold or the flu, but they stay much longer. Some of the common symptoms include chest pain, fever, cough, vomiting, and shortness of breath. Hence, early diagnosis is preferred for the proper treatment of pneumonia. There are various methods for diagnosing pneumonia like CT scan, MRI, and chest X-ray, out of which X-ray imaging is the most cost-effective and clinically proven procedure [2].

4.1.1 ARTIFICIAL INTELLIGENCE

Traditionally, medical experts evaluate lung infection based on their judgment and the method of treatment to cure the infection. This will take a lot of time and sometimes the level of disease may appear unclear. Various computer-assisted procedures are available to efficiently predict lung disease and its infection rate using chest X-rays [3, 4].

Machine Learning (ML) and Deep Learning (DL) models can be incorporated to predict lung infection using X-ray images. ML can be defined as the study of computer algorithms designed for automation, learning from its experience. ML is a subset of Artificial intelligence (AI), it tries to mimic the human brain. There are two kinds of ML approaches, i.e., Supervised Learning and Unsupervised Learning [5].

Deep Learning, on the other hand, is a subset of machine learning and can be defined as an artificial neural network with one or more hidden layers (in addition to the input and output layers) that can enhance system performance in terms of accuracy [6]. DL algorithms can be very useful for problems involving feature extraction and classification. The prediction accuracy of a DL model is typically better than that of an ML model. Therefore, their performance in various fields and rapid advancements are widely utilized in different domains such as healthcare [7].

This study focuses on object detection for predicting pneumonia in human lungs. Object detection is a computer vision task used to identify and locate multiple objects. Object detection, as opposed to simple classification, offers a more comprehensive understanding of the object as a whole with a bounding box. Each object possesses certain features, and object detection techniques utilize these features to distinguish between them. Object detection can enhance the efficiency of various processes and reduce human effort. There are several deep learning approaches employed for object detection. Algorithms like Single Shot Detector (SSD), Region-Based Convolutional Neural Network (R-CNN), and You Only Look Once (YOLO) use Convolutional Neural Network (CNN) to detect objects in an image [8]. The advantage of utilizing a deep learning-based object detection approach is that the entire detection process is carried out without explicitly identifying the features to be used for data classification.

4.1.2 R-CNN

R-CNN model uses a selective search algorithm to detect objects. In this algorithm, many regions are generated and checked for having objects. R-CNN works in a way to classify and localize objects with a bounding box [9]. There are various object detection models under R-CNN like Fast R-CNN and Faster R-CNN. This R-CNN method focuses more on dividing an image into different parts and then predicting the result based on the part with a higher probability of containing an object. Fast R-CNN utilizes deep ConvNets, which is a fast framework for the classification and detection of objects in a frame.

Faster R-CNN, on the other hand, uses a Region Proposal Network (RPN) instead of a Selective search algorithm. RPN is a single unified network for object detection. Some of the applications of Faster R-CNN include image captioning, 3-D object detection, and many more. Mask R-CNN helps locate every object's exact pixel rather than just making a bounding box. This task can be performed by adding a branch to Faster R-CNN; this branch is responsible for providing a binary output known as a mask.

This study focuses on implementing the Mask R-CNN methodology for Pneumonia detection using X-ray images of human lungs. This can be very useful for detecting pneumonia in human lungs. Hence, early treatment can be done. The study is further categorized as follows: Section 4.2 highlights the related research work previously done in this field. Section 4.3 discusses the dataset and methodology adopted to carry out this study. Results obtained in this study are discussed in Section 4.4. Finally, the conclusion and future directions of this study are covered in Section 4.5.

4.2 LITERATURE SURVEY

Disease detection and diagnosis have been active areas of research for several decades. The healthcare sector is one of the important sectors, shifting from hospital-centric and reactive to a personalized and preventive system. This demands a more intelligent procedure. There are many advances in deep learning that have played an effective role in the medical field. Many researchers are adopting different object detection methodologies to develop a more efficient system.

Bhandary et al. proposed a modified DL model to detect lung abnormalities. They used chest X-ray and lung CT-scan images in their study [1]. The model uses AlexNet with an SVM classifier and achieves a classification accuracy of 86.47%. They also concluded that DL techniques offer better accuracy. Sousa et al. deployed three machine learning classifiers to detect and classify pneumonia on radiograph images [2]. Their Support Vector Machine (accuracy of 77%), K-Nearest Neighbors (accuracy of 70%), and Naïve Bayes Classifier (accuracy of 68%) are optimized with the best features to ensure there is no overfitting. Rajpurkar et al. developed CheXNeXt, a convolutional neural network used to detect 14 different pathologies using chest radiographs, including pneumonia and pulmonary masses. Their ChestX-ray8 dataset contains 420 images, with at least 50 cases of each of the original pathology labels [3].

Varshni et al. proposed a combination of CNN-based feature extraction and supervised classifier, predicting whether the patient got pneumonia or not. Also, they applied transfer learning algorithms, out of which SVM with DenseNet-169 as feature extractor gave desired result of Area Under Curve (AUC) as 0.8002 [11]. SSD RetinaNet pre-trained on ImageNet was used on data for 25,684 patients. Models took a much longer time to converge but after pre-training, it works better. The model achieved 87.5% of predicting a bounding box. Their results largely depend on thresholds [12].

A similar approach for automatic detection of pneumonia and classification between viral and bacterial pneumonia from X-ray images was carried out. The authors had used four different pre-trained CNN models: AlexNet, ResNet18, SqueezeNet, and DenseNet201 for transfer learning. Around 5,247 images of chest X-rays including 3 classes (normal, viral, and bacterial) were preprocessed and then trained for classification based on transfer learning. The study had three schemes: normal vs pneumonia (accuracy 98%), viral vs bacterial pneumonia (accuracy 95%), and normal vs bacterial vs viral pneumonia (accuracy 93.3%) [13].

Toğaçar et al. utilized some of the pre-trained CNN models (AlexNet, VGG16, and VGG19) and improved classification accuracy of the prediction model for two different classes (Normal and Pneumonia). One of the disadvantages of this procedure was that the preprocessing of pneumonia images was not considered by the researchers [14].

Tilve et al. proposed a two-step Pneumonia detection technique. Image preprocessing was done in the first step, a pre-trained model was deployed in the second step. They provided an in-depth survey paper comparing various techniques like CNN, ResNet, and ANN. In addition to that, they also focused on image preprocessing methods to convert raw X-ray images into standard formats that can be further used for analysis and detection [15].

Hashmi et al. proposed a novel approach combining some supervised deep learning approaches including InceptionV3, MobileNetV3, DenseNet121, and ResNet18. In addition to this, they used transfer learning to fine-tune the deep learning models for getting higher accuracy. AUC score was 99.76 on unseen data [16]. Zhang et al. proposed a Confidence Aware Anomaly Detection (CAAD) Model, a combination of a confidence prediction module, an anomaly detection module, and a feature extractor. This CAD model performs binary classification on a clinical X-viral dataset, which includes 5,997 viral pneumonia cases and 37,393 healthy cases. They observed that anomaly detection works well with the binary classification model on chest X-ray images. False negatives can be reduced by learning model confidence to predict failures. The model achieved an AUC of 83.61% and a sensitivity of 71.70% on the unseen COVID dataset [17]. A customized VGG19 model was proposed to detect pneumonia on chest radiograph images. AlexNet, ResNet50, VGG16, and

VGG19 architectures were used in this research, out of which VGG19 with SoftMax gave the desired results [19].

Yu et al. developed a deep learning framework that classified the X-ray images, CGNet. This CGNet framework included 3 main components: feature extractor, graph-based feature reconstruction, and classification task. They used transfer learning to train the CNN model to classify and also to produce features. Then features were combined with the help of graph-based feature reconstruction. At last, GNet, a shallow neural network was used to combine features as input and classify between normal and pneumonia on chest radiographs [20].

Kundu et al. developed an ensemble framework to build a weighted average ensemble that considers the result obtained from three different CNN models, i.e., ResNet18, DenseNet121, and GoogLeNet. A five-fold cross-validation scheme was used in their study. They used the RSNA challenge dataset and obtained 86.86% accuracy with a precision rate of 86.89%, a sensitivity of 87.02%, and an F1-score of 86.95% [21].

Chagas et al. proposed a real-time Internet of Things (IoT) framework to identify diseases via chest radiographs. The research study consisted of 12 different frameworks of CNN that were trained on ImageNet to operate as feature extractors. Simultaneously, learning methods like Naïve Bayes, Multilayer Perceptron (MLP), and Random Forest were combined with CNN. Also, Chagas et al. concluded that the VGG19 framework with SVM classifier outperforms the other models in detecting pneumonia. Another advantage of their research was the availability of an IoT system, which enabled the insertion of X-ray images and produced real-time accurate results [23].

Yao et al. proposed an improved framework based on faster R-CNN for pneumonia detection. It was a low residual dilated bottleneck neural network structure known as DeepConv-DilatedNet, which was used as a foundation for a 2-stage detector utilizing faster R-CNN. In addition to this, the Soft-NMS algorithm was used to ensure the quality and filter the anchor box. To improve localization accuracy, anchor boxes were generated with the help of the k-means++ algorithm. They obtained a Mean Average Precision (mAP) of 39.23% on the RSNA dataset using convolutional neural networks [24].

Chakraborthy et al. built a model having 17 layers, including three convolutional layers, five dense layers, and one output layer. Several max-pooling layers had been added to the design to reduce dimensionality. The constructed model had a 95.62% accuracy rate, with recall and precision rates of 95% and 96%, respectively [26]. Shah et al. presented a systematic review of different deep learning models used for the classification of pneumonia. Five datasets including X-ray images and CT scans were taken into consideration for research work [27]. However, most studies performed only classification tasks; there was no algorithm to detect and locate the infected area. There are very few research studies that utilize object detection techniques, and those that do have less accuracy. This study will provide a reliable object detection algorithm for accurately detecting and specifying the region on X-ray images.

4.3 METHODOLOGY

This section contains the description of the dataset, a prelude to an acquired methodology for the research work. The research work employs a specific type of DL method that can be applied in pneumonia detection systems to classify and detect unhealthy individuals. To obtain this, we have used the Mask R-CNN method as the pneumonia detection technique. Google Collaboratory using Python version 3.7.10 is used to implement this research study.

4.3.1 DATASET

RSNA Dataset: This dataset has been published by the Radiological Society of North America (RSNA). The dataset is being preserved and made freely available for the scientific community to use. This dataset includes 26,684 samples and is a subset of a larger dataset created by the National Institute of Health (NIH). The RSNA dataset in the training set contains 26,684 samples with three types of labels: lung opacity (6,012), no lung opacity/not normal (11,821), and normal (8,851).

This includes both the samples for males and females. In addition to this, the dataset also contains 3,000 sample images, which can be used to test the proposed method. All these samples are in the form of DICOM images. Although the RSNA dataset is part of the NIH dataset, the two datasets have many distinctions. The RSNA dataset was created primarily for pneumonia cases and provides crucial and reliable information for disease classification and detection [28] (Figure 4.1).

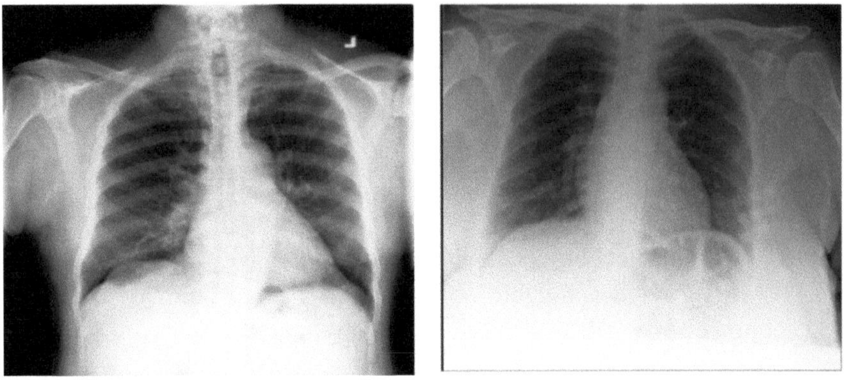

FIGURE 4.1 Sample dataset.

Source: Reprinted from RSNA pneumonia detection challenge.(n.d.). Copyright. RSNA

4.3.2 PROPOSED METHODOLOGY

The main objective of Region-Based Convolutional Network (R-CNN) is to solve the problem of object detection. Mask R-CNN can be considered as the extension of Faster R-CNN, but Faster R-CNN has class labels and a bounding box offset. Mask R-CNN has a third parameter known as the object mask. It takes the CNN feature map as an input and outputs a binary mask. A binary mask is a matrix that produces 1s for locations where that pixel belongs to the object and gives 0s for other locations. The additional mask output differs from the class and box outputs as it requires a finer spatial arrangement of an object to be extracted. The pixel-to-pixel alignment, which is the main missing piece of Faster R-CNN, is a critical component of Mask R-CNN.

Mask R-CNN uses the two-stage technique, with the first stage (which is RPN). Mask R-CNN outputs a binary mask for each Region of Interest (RoI) in the second stage and predicts the class and box offset. To implement the object detection methodology, the dataset is first analyzed by doing the exploratory data analysis. There are a total of 30,277 X-ray images with 3 different classes in DCM format present in the dataset shown in Figure 4.2.

In this study, the weights of the pre-trained Mask R-CNN model are modified according to the requirements. The model was first trained on some common dataset, then the model is trained on the RSNA Pneumonia detection dataset. The whole process of object detection is divided into two steps. Mask R-CNN generates the object proposal in the first stage,

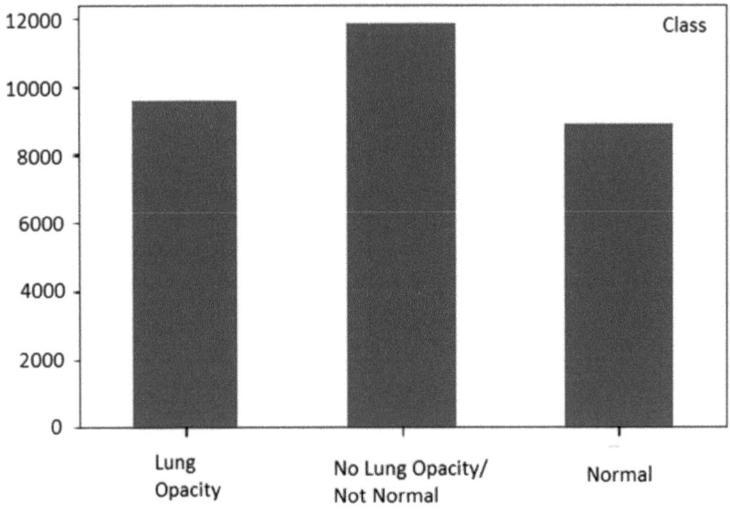

FIGURE 4.2 Detailed class information.

which classifies whether the object has a region of interest or not, i.e., background or foreground. Classifying the object class, generating the bounding box, and generation of masks for the objects is done in the second stage. Mask R-CNN utilizes the ResNet 50 architecture to train the model. A deep neural network architecture, ResNet 50 has 50 layers that utilize residual learning [35]. Residual blocks are used to connect the input of one layer to the output of the next layer. One of the main advantages of a residual layer is that we can skip some of the layers without affecting the prediction accuracy. Using this, the model tries to make a bounding box around the region where the lung opacity is found. Then in the testing phase, the model itself predicts the bounding region for pneumonia.

Figure 4.3 shows the proposed methodology for the research study. In this first the type of data is analyzed, then it is converted to a machine-understandable format for processing under the Mask R-CNN technique.

4.4 RESULTS

This section focuses on discussing the main findings of the research work. The prediction of pneumonia is divided into two steps. First, the model is trained with training data having all three classes, i.e., normal, abnormal, and pneumonia. Also, the dataset contains lung images of both male and

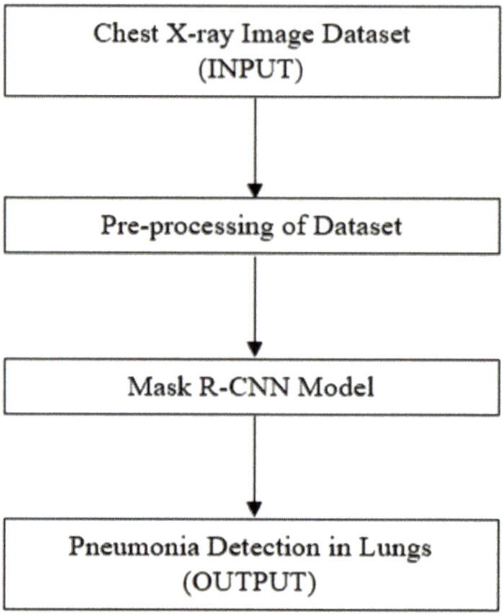

FIGURE 4.3 Proposed methodology.

female patients. Firstly, the 2 gender classes are distinguished. Figure 4.4 elaborates the total number of each class in the training set.

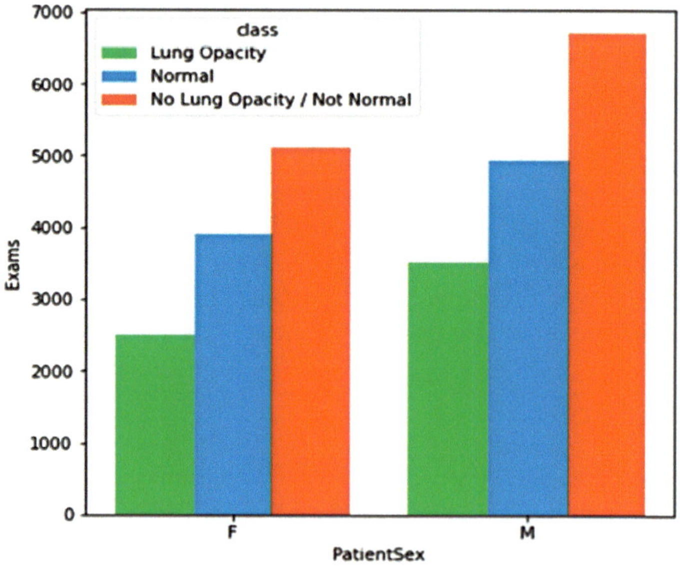

FIGURE 4.4 Patient sex and class.

By analyzing the training set in terms of patient gender, the model creates a bounding box around the infected area. The bounding box will denote the lung opacity on chest X-ray images. It has been found that the maximum number of bounding boxes that occur on an image is 4. The Mask R-CNN model shows very good accuracy in detecting pneumonia in X-ray images by predicting and creating a bounding box around the infected area. The results are shown in Figure 4.5 as classifying and detecting pneumonia.

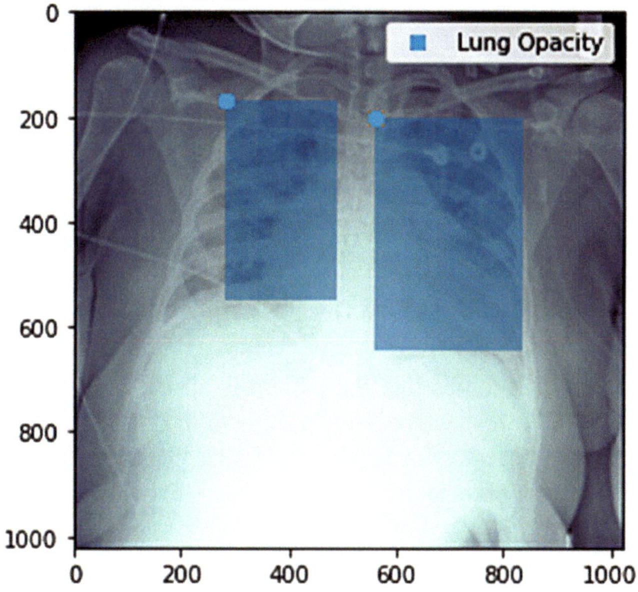

FIGURE 4.5 Lung opacities.

Figure 4.5 shows the results obtained from a dataset where the patient has pneumonia in one of the lungs. It is observed that in many cases, pneumonia occurs in both lungs. However, there are instances where the object detection model detects pneumonia in only one of the lungs. A maximum of 4 bounding boxes are observed to locate pneumonia. With good precision, the model also classifies normal and abnormal (no lung opacity) X-ray images. There are cases where the model predicts no opacity, but the X-ray image shows some abnormalities. In other words, the X-ray image shows no sign of pneumonia, but there are some abnormalities present as shown in Figure 4.6.

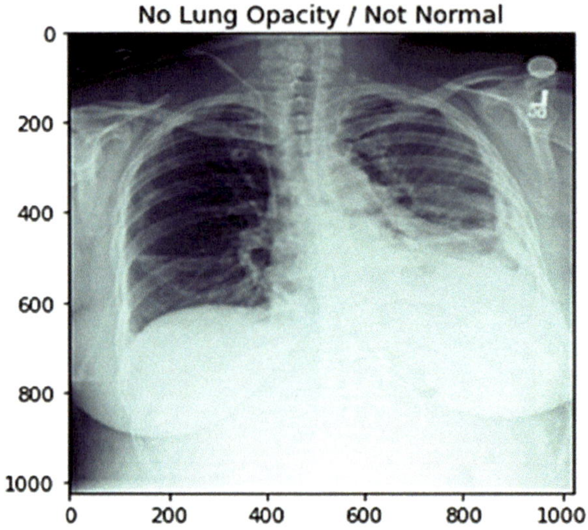

FIGURE 4.6 Abnormality in lungs.

Normal class specifies that the patient is absolutely fine, i.e., there is no problem in their respective X-ray as shown in Figure 4.7. It is observed that the model possesses an accuracy of 93.88% in predicting the right class with bounding boxes.

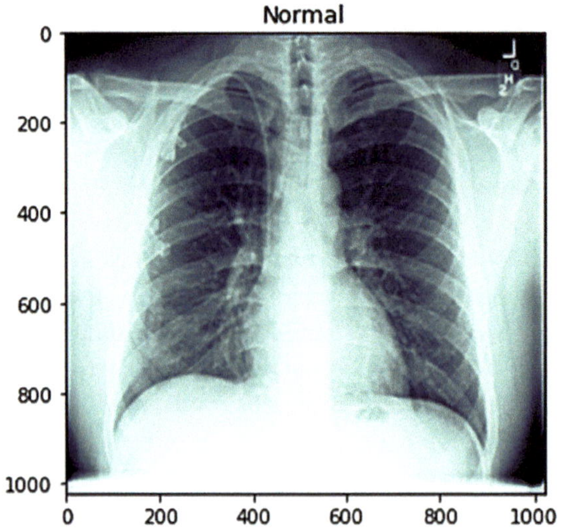

FIGURE 4.7 Normal lungs.

4.5 CONCLUSION

It is very important to detect and diagnose pneumonia in the early stages. This research chapter focuses on providing a reliable pneumonia detection model that takes X-ray images of human lungs and based on certain features will predict whether the person is suffering from pneumonia or not. In addition to that, it will also detect the location or region where the infection occurs. In other words, it will localize the lung opacities region. The model is based on the Mask R-CNN method, ResNet-50 is used as the backbone of the model. We have used the RSNA dataset for the study. Since the dataset is in DCM format, it is converted into a well-understandable format (.png) to perform certain operations before feeding it to the model. Around 26,684 X-ray images have been trained on our model, then it is used as the object detection model. The model achieves 93.88% accuracy in detecting the lung opacity regions.

This research can further be extended to different datasets that require the method of detection. Data Augmentation can be added to improve the model performance. The proposed method can be applied to the development of high-performance computer-aided diagnosis systems for additional medical imaging applications. Since the model is built upon the features of deep learning (RCNN), transfer learning on some state-of-the-art CNN architectures like SSD, YOLO, etc., can be utilized to improve the performance measures.

KEYWORDS

- **deep learning**
- **healthcare**
- **lung opacity**
- **mask R-CNN**
- **object detection**
- **pneumonia detection**
- **Radiological Society of North America**
- **region proposal network**
- **X-ray images**

REFERENCES

1. Bhandary, A., Prabhu, G. A., Rajinikanth, V., Thanaraj, K. P., Satapathy, S. C., Robbins, D. E., Shasky, C., Zhang, Y.-D., Tavares, J. M. R. S., & Raja, N. S. M. (2020). Deep-learning framework to detect lung abnormality – A study with chest X-ray and lung CT scan images. *Pattern Recognition Letters, 129*, 271–278. https://doi.org/10.1016/j.patrec.2019.11.013.
2. Sousa, R. T., Marques, O., Soares, F. A. A. M. N., Sene, I. I. G., Jr., de Oliveira, L. L. G., & Spoto, E. S. (2013). Comparative performance analysis of machine learning classifiers in detection of childhood pneumonia using chest radiographs. *Procedia Computer Science, 18*, 2579–2582. https://doi.org/10.1016/j.procs.2013.05.444.
3. Rajpurkar, P., Irvin, J., Ball, R. L., Zhu, K., Yang, B., Mehta, H., Duan, T., Ding, D., Bagul, A., Langlotz, C. P., Patel, B. N., Yeom, K. W., Shpanskaya, K., Blankenberg, F. G., Seekins, J., Amrhein, T. J., Mong, D. A., Halabi, S. S., Zucker, E. J., Ng, A. Y., & Lungren, M. P. (2018). Deep learning for chest radiograph diagnosis: A retrospective comparison of the CheXNeXt algorithm to practicing radiologists. *PLOS Medicine, 15*(11), e1002686. https://doi.org/10.1371/journal.pmed.1002686.
4. Irvin, J., Rajpurkar, P., Ko, M., Yu, Y., Ciurea-Ilcus, S., Chute, C., Marklund, H., Haghgoo, B., Ball, R., Shpanskaya, K., Seekins, J., Mong, D. A., Halabi, S. S., Sandberg, J. K., Jones, R., Larson, D. B., Langlotz, C. P., Patel, B. N., Lungren, M. P., & Ng, A. Y. (2019). CheXpert: A large chest radiograph dataset with uncertainty labels and expert comparison. *Proceedings of the AAAI Conference on Artificial Intelligence, 33*(01), 590–597. https://doi.org/10.1609/aaai.v33i01.3301590.
5. Siddique, S., & Chow, J. C. L. (2021). Machine learning in healthcare communication. *Encyclopedia, 1*(1), 220–239. https://doi.org/10.3390/encyclopedia1010021.
6. Deng, L. (2014). Deep learning: Methods and applications. *Foundations and Trends in Signal Processing, 7*(3–4), 197–387. https://doi.org/10.1561/2000000039.
7. Shamshirband, S., Fathi, M., Dehzangi, A., Chronopoulos, A. T., & Alinejad-Rokny, H. (2021). A review on deep learning approaches in healthcare systems: Taxonomies, challenges, and open issues. *Journal of Biomedical Informatics, 113*, 103627. https://doi.org/10.1016/j.jbi.2020.103627.
8. Nallanti, M., Venkateswara Rao, P. (2022). A review on object detection in the healthcare using deep learning techniques. *International Journal of Engineering Applied Sciences and Technology, 6*(7), 159–166. Retrieved from: https://www.ijeast.com/papers/159-166,Tesma607,IJEAST.pdf (accessed on 31 May 2024).
9. Girshick, R., Donahue, J., Darrell, T., & Malik, J. (2013). Rich feature hierarchies for accurate object detection and semantic segmentation. arXiv. 2014, eprint (1311.2524), https://doi.org/10.48550/arXiv.1311.2524.
10. Zhao, W., Luo, X., & Qiu, T. (2017). Smart healthcare. *Applied Sciences, 7*(11), 1176. https://doi.org/10.3390/app7111176.
11. Varshni, D., Thakral, K., Agarwal, L., Nijhawan, R., & Mittal, A. (2019). Pneumonia detection using CNN based feature extraction. In *2019 IEEE International Conference on Electrical, Computer and Communication Technologies (ICECCT)* (pp. 1–7). IEEE. https://doi.org/10.1109/ICECCT.2019.8869364.

12. Gabruseva, T., Poplavskiy, D., & Kalinin, A. A. (2020). Deep learning for automatic pneumonia detection. arXiv. https://arxiv.org/abs/2001.11038, DOI:10.1109/CVPRW50498.2020.00183.
13. Rahman, T., Chowdhury, M. E. H., Khandakar, A., Islam, K. R., Islam, K. F., Mahbub, Z. B., Kadir, M. A., & Kashem, S. (2020). Transfer learning with deep convolutional neural network (CNN) for pneumonia detection using chest X-ray. *Applied Sciences, 10*(9), 3233. https://doi.org/10.3390/app10093233.
14. Toğaçar, M., Ergen, B., Cömert, Z., & Özyurt, F. (2020). A deep feature learning model for pneumonia detection applying a combination of MRMR feature selection and machine learning models. *IRBM, 41*(4), 212–222. https://doi.org/10.1016/j.irbm.2019.10.006.
15. Tilve, A., Nayak, S., Vernekar, S., Turi, D., & Shetgaonkar, P. R. (2020). Pneumonia detection using deep learning approaches. In *2020 International Conference on Emerging Trends in Information Technology and Engineering* (ic-ETITE). *IEEE.* https://doi.org/10.1109/ic-ETITE47903.2020.334. DOI: https://doi.org/10.46647/ijetms.2023.v07i02.082.
16. Hashmi, M. F., Katiyar, S., Keskar, A. G., Bokde, N. D., & Geem, Z. W. (2020). Efficient pneumonia detection in chest X-ray images using deep transfer learning. *Diagnostics, 10*(6), 417. https://doi.org/10.3390/diagnostics10060417.
17. Zhang, J., Xie, Y., Pang, G., Liao, Z., Verjans, J., Li, W., Sun, Z., He, J., Li, Y., Shen, C., & Xia, Y. (2021). Viral pneumonia screening on chest X-rays using confidence-aware anomaly detection. *IEEE Transactions on Medical Imaging, 40*(3), 879–890. https://doi.org/10.1109/TMI.2020.3040950.
18. Pan, I., Cadrin-Chênevert, A., & Cheng, P. M. (2019). Tackling the Radiological Society of North America pneumonia detection challenge. *AJR American Journal of Roentgenology, 213*(3), 568–574. https://doi.org/10.2214/AJR.19.21512.
19. Dey, N., Zhang, Y. D., Rajinikanth, V., Pugalenthi, R., & Raja, N. S. M. (2021). Customized VGG19 architecture for pneumonia detection in chest X-rays. *Pattern Recognition Letters, 143*, 67–74. https://doi.org/10.1016/j.patrec.2020.12.010.
20. Yu, X., Wang, S. H., & Zhang, Y. D. (2021). CGNet: A graph-knowledge embedded convolutional neural network for detection of pneumonia. *Information Processing & Management, 58*(1), 102411. https://doi.org/10.1016/j.ipm.2020.102411.
21. Kundu, R., Das, R., Geem, Z. W., Han, G. T., & Sarkar, R. (2021). Pneumonia detection in chest X-ray images using an ensemble of deep learning models. *PLoS One, 16*(9), e0256630. https://doi.org/10.1371/journal.pone.0256630.
22. Gilbert, D. N., Leggett, J. E., Wang, L., Ferdosian, S., Gelfer, G. D., Johnston, M. L., Footer, B. W., Hendrickson, K. W., Park, H. S., White, E. E., & Heffner, J. (2021). Enhanced detection of community-acquired pneumonia pathogens with the BioFire® Pneumonia FilmArray® Panel. *Diagnostic Microbiology and Infectious Disease, 99*(3), 115246. https://doi.org/10.1016/j.diagmicrobio.2020.115246.
23. Chagas, J. V. S. das, de A Rodrigues, D., Ivo, R. F., Hassan, M. M., de Albuquerque, V. H. C., & Filho, P. P. R. (2021). A new approach for the detection of pneumonia in children using CXR images based on a real-time IoT system. *Journal of Real-Time Image Processing, 18*(4), 1099–1114. https://doi.org/10.1007/s11554-021-01086-y.

24. Yao, S., Chen, Y., Tian, X., & Jiang, R. (2021). Pneumonia detection using an improved algorithm based on Faster R-CNN. *Computational and Mathematical Methods in Medicine, 2021*, 8854892. https://doi.org/10.1155/2021/8854892.
25. Sharma, N., Bhushan, B., Kaushik, I., & Debnath, N. C. (2021). Applicability of blockchain technology in healthcare industry: Applications, challenges, and solutions. In *Internet of Things* (pp. 339–370). Springer International Publishing. https://doi.org/10.1007/978-3-030-66633-0_15.
26. Chakraborty, S., Aich, S., Sim, J. S., & Kim, H. C. (2019). Detection of pneumonia from chest X-rays using a convolutional neural network architecture. *International Conference on Future Information & Communication Engineering, 11*(1), 98–102.
27. Shah, A., & Shah, M. (2022). Advancement of deep learning in pneumonia/COVID-19 classification and localization: A systematic review with qualitative and quantitative analysis. *Chronic Diseases and Translational Medicine, 8*(3), 149–243. DOI: https://doi.org/10.1002/cdt3.17.
28. RSNA pneumonia detection challenge. (n.d.). Retrieved from: https://www.kaggle.com/competitions/rsna-pneumonia-detection-challenge/overview (accessed on 31 May 2024).
29. Tiwari, R., Sharma, N., Kaushik, I., Tiwari, A., & Bhushan, B. (2019). Evolution of IoT & data analytics using deep learning. In 2019 International Conference on Computing, Communication, and Intelligent Systems (ICCCIS). *IEEE Proceedings*, pp. 418–423, https://doi.org/10.1109/ICCCIS48478.2019.8974481.
30. Harjani, M., Grover, M., Sharma, N., & Kaushik, I. (2019). "Analysis of Various Machine Learning Algorithm for Cardiac Pulse Prediction," *2019 International Conference on Computing, Communication, and Intelligent Systems (ICCCIS), Greater Noida, India, 2019*, pp. 244–249, DOI: 10.1109/ICCCIS48478.2019.8974519.
31. Sharma, A., Sharma, N., Kaushik, I., Kumar, S., & Khatoon, N. (2020). Predictive analysis of type 2 diabetes using hybrid ML model and IoT. In *IoT Security Paradigms and Applications* (pp. 303–320). CRC Press. https://doi.org/10.1201/9781003054115-14.
32. Sharma, N., Kaushik, I., Rathi, R., & Kumar, S. (2020). Evaluation of accidental death records using hybrid genetic algorithm. *SSRN Electronic Journal, 3*, 1–6. https://doi.org/10.2139/ssrn.3563084.
33. Varshney, T., Chug, A., & Singh, A. P. (2021). Deep learning models for prediction of tomato powdery mildew disease. In *2021 8th International Conference on Signal Processing and Integrated Networks (SPIN) Proceedings*, pp. 1036–1041, electronicISSN:2688–769X, Print on Demand (PoD) ISSN: 2688–7681.
34. Sharma, N., Kaushik, I., Bhushan, B., Gautam, S., & Khamparia, A. (2020). Applicability of WSN and biometric models in the field of healthcare. In *Deep Learning Strategies for Security Enhancement in Wireless Sensor Networks* (pp. 304–329). IGI Global. https://doi.org/10.4018/978-1-7998-5068-7.ch016.
35. Karacı, A. (2022). VGGCOV19-NET: Automatic detection of COVID-19 cases from X-ray images using modified VGG19 CNN architecture and YOLO algorithm. *Neural Computing and Applications, 34(10), 1–22.* https://doi.org/10.1007/s00521-022-06918-x.

36. He, K., Zhang, X., Ren, S., & Sun, J. (2016). Deep residual learning for image recognition. In *2016 IEEE Conference on Computer Vision and Pattern Recognition (CVPR). IEEE proceedings*, pp. 770–778. DOI: https://arxiv.org/pdf/1512.03385.pdf.
37. Jaiswal, A. K., Tiwari, P., Kumar, S., Gupta, D., Khanna, A., & Rodrigues, J. J. P. C. (2019). Identifying pneumonia in chest X-rays: A deep learning approach. *Measurement, 145*, 511–518. https://doi.org/10.1016/j.measurement.2019.05.076.
38. Lecrosnier, L., Khemmar, R., Ragot, N., Decoux, B., Rossi, R., Kefi, N., & Ertaud, J. Y. (2020). Deep learning-based object detection, localization and tracking for smart wheelchair healthcare mobility. *International Journal of Environmental Research and Public Health, 18*(1), 91. https://doi.org/10.3390/ijerph18010091.
39. R, E., V, S., V, V., & Mahanti, A. (2021). Cervical cancer diagnostics healthcare system using hybrid object detection adversarial networks. *IEEE Journal of Biomedical and Health Informatics*, PP, 1–1. https://doi.org/10.1109/JBHI.2021.3094311.
40. Goyal, S., Sharma, N., Bhushan, B., Shankar, A., & Sagayam, M. (2021). IoT enabled technology in secured healthcare: Applications, challenges and future directions. In *Cognitive Internet of Medical Things for Smart Healthcare* (pp. 25–48). Springer International Publishing. https://doi.org/10.1007/978-3-030-55833-8_2.
41. Darapaneni, N., Ranjan, A., Bright, D., Trivedi, D., Kumar, K., Kumar, V., & Paduri, A. R. (2022). Pneumonia detection in chest X-rays using neural networks. arXiv., eprint={2204.03618}, pp. 1–21, https://doi.org/10.48550/ARXIV.2204.03618.
42. Makhanov, N., Tu, N. A., & Wong, K. S. (2022). A survey on deep learning advances and emerging issues in pneumonia and COVID-19 prediction. In *2022 IEEE International Conference on Big Data and Smart Computing (BigComp). IEEE Proceedings*, pp. 96–103. https://doi.org/10.1109/. BigComp54360.2022.00029.
43. Bodapati, J. D., & Rohith, V. N. (2022). ChxCapsNet: Deep capsule network with transfer learning for evaluating pneumonia in paediatric chest radiographs. *Measurement, 188*, 110491. https://doi.org/10.1016/j.measurement.2021.110491.

CHAPTER 5

Corona Tracker: An Application for Monitoring and Tracking the Corona Disease

SHAILENDRA SINGH GAUR, JAI GAUR, and VANSH GUPTA

Department of IT, Bhagwan Parshuram Institute of Technology, Delhi, India

ABSTRACT

More intriguing features, such as disease prediction based on symptoms and guidance for next steps, such as finding a suitable doctor in the user's area, will greatly enhance this program. This chapter gives the details of the application developed using ReactJS and some basic front-end development techniques for tracking Corona by monitoring the user.

5.1 INTRODUCTION

'Corona tracker' is a useful application with a bunch of exciting features that it offers to the users from page reloads to all coronavirus-related data under a single web page. It covers all scenarios to achieve the requirements of any user searching for worldwide or country-wise details regarding coronavirus. This Application is developed for serving its users to the fullest of its potential by providing them a platform where they can get the data and information about the coronavirus not only worldwide but also country-wise and in graphical as well as geographical display. Though the application is based more on the front-end development, dynamic data is also given equal preference. The data is collected by asynchronous API

Data-Driven Analytics for Healthcare: Artificial Intelligence and Machine Learning for Medical Diagnostics. Meghna Sharma, Priyanka Vashisht, A. V. Senthil Kumar, Chitra Singh, and Abdelmalek Amine (Eds.)

calls disease. That provides dynamic data depending on the endpoint used during the call. In simple words, disease.sh acts as a server to which we make GET requests to provide an endpoint and according to the endpoint, it gives JSON data in response.

5.2 RELATED WORK

In the world of web development, ReactJS is a far superior technique for representing data. And for any data analyst, how the data is represented by the user is crucial.

It is more convenient for the user if it can gather all information from a single source and do it with only a few mouse clicks. In medical research, data analysis and visualization are essential tools for analyzing and conveying findings, particularly in epidemiological surveillance [3].

Many government agencies, universities, and companies have launched applications that help analyze real-time situations or viruses by providing updates about the number of coronavirus cases in our surroundings [2] so that conclusions could be made about how to protect us from its widespread effects.

The AarogyaSetu application in India and the COVID Symptom Study in the UK are some of the applications provided by the governments of their respective countries to track the contacts of people in their surroundings and the current situation of COVID-19, such that the chain of cause could be easily detected, and its transmission is reduced to an extent by executing plans made with data in consideration.

These are apps that track COVID-19 and require high-priority GPS and Bluetooth permissions to track the spread of infection and give an idea of how close you are to an infected person, and in which zone you spend your time, calculating your risks of being infected. When considered in the field of research on healthcare these days, coronavirus has become one of the most important topics of research and development.

Before representing any kind of coronavirus data, its authenticity is everything, and fetching the right data requires good knowledge of some JS features. Analysis is something that helps reduce errors and make things precise, but it does so only when done on correct data.

React JS, as a frontend library, can help write code in components so that everything you see on the web is a component that makes code reusable. Whenever any change is required somewhere, the whole code need not be touched, and the part that needs an update can be easily modified. From writing reusable components to a virtual DOM, it has features that can help not only in the perfect representation of data but also in the fast execution of changes on the screen.

It can easily be integrated with REDUX as a store and Firebase as a database. React JS is one of the biggest fields of development these days and is being used by big MNCs for UI development.

Thus, the use of this kind of technology may help create a wonderful UI that helps users to see COVID-19 related data on a single web page with minimal interactions or clicks, boosting the process of analyzers who analyze the data to find perfect solutions. An alarming situation requires an alarming solution, so using ReactJS as a technology can make the interface faster and represent the data fully on a single page with minimal user intervention.

It covers all scenarios to meet the requirements of any user searching for worldwide or country-wise details regarding coronavirus. This application is developed to serve its users to the fullest potential by providing them a platform where they can access data and information about coronavirus globally and on a country level, displayed graphically and geographically.

Figure 5.1 shows how the whole website is converted into different components, with components at the top of the UI tree being parent components and components below parents being child components.

In React, all the properties of a parent component can be passed to a child component by passing key-value pairs to the child component when called inside the parent component.

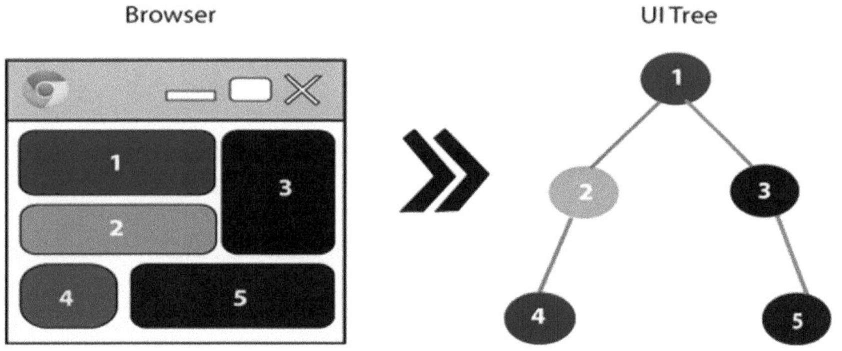

FIGURE 5.1 React JS–DOM and its components.

5.3 ABOUT REACTJS

Facebook created ReactJS, a component-based JavaScript library. It was open-sourced by Facebook in 2013 and has been received with enthusiasm by a large developer community. Netflix, Yahoo!, GitHub, and Codecademy are among the early adopters in the corporate world.

Devs have praised react for its:

- Performance;
- Flexibility;
- Declarative, component-based approach to UI.

React was created with the demands of Facebook's development team in mind, and it's especially well-suited to complicated web apps with a lot of user interaction and dynamic data.

5.3.1 REACTJS USES

- The creation of dynamic web applications is easier.
- It increases productivity and helps in maintenance.
- Ensures faster rendering of virtual DOM.
- It ensures to have a stable code.
- Flux and Redux architecture.
- It has SEO friendly features.
- A helpful developer toolset.
- It is used by most Fortune 500 companies.
- React native is great for mobile application development.
- Easy to learn.

5.3.2 VIRTUAL DOM?

The DOM contains UI components such as elements and attributes (document object model). Virtual DOM is a memory-light clone of the real DOM, consisting of a node tree listing of components.

It is created by the render() function in ReactJS.A new virtual DOM is constructed every time the underlying data changes, with previous virtual DOM differences compared and just the changes updated in the actual DOM. ReactDOM.Render() differs from ReactDOM in that it only updates DOM items that have changed.

5.3.3 JAVASCRIPT JSX?

- The JavaScript XML extension isn't browser-readable JavaScript. It's a JavaScript file that includes JavaScript XML code, which is like HTML, and it must be compiled before being transmitted to a web browser, which is done using a JavaScript XML compiler.
- JSX elements are regarded like JavaScript expressions and can be saved as variables, supplied to functions, or stored in objects or arrays.
- There must be precisely one outermost element in every JSX expression. JSX expressions are usually wrapped in a div.
- Rendering a JSX element is bringing it to life on the screen. This is how we render JSX expressions:
- The ReactDOM library is a JavaScript library.
- The word class is commonly used as an attribute name in HTML; however, it is not allowed in JSX. Instead, we must use className. Because class is a reserved term in JavaScript, and JavaScript XML is converted to JavaScript.
- In HTML, the forward slash is optional for self-closing tags such as img, input, br, but it is not in JS XML.
- The period of a JavaScript expression is indicated by curly brackets.

5.3.4 COMPONENT

A component is a short computer program that performs a specific purpose and may be reused. Most of the time, it was to render HTML. We may utilize several JSX components. The render method must include all variables and conditions. 'this' refers to the object that this enclosing method is applied upon. A React app can include dozens, if not hundreds, of components that interact with one another. Using an import statement when you're attempting to import variables from a file other than the current one isn't nearly enough.

5.3.5 LIFECYCLE METHODS

During the lifecycle of a React component, lifecycle methods are invoked. When a component is mounted, it automatically invokes the following three lifecycle methods:

1. **Component WillMount:** It is called just before render when a component is rendered for the first time.

2. **Render:** We'd been talking about it the whole time.

3. **ComponentDidMount:** As soon as the HTML from the render has completed loading for a component, componentDidMount is called.

If your React application makes use of AJAX to get initial data from an API, then componentDidMount is the location where the AJAX request should be made. SetTimeout and setInterval are useful for connecting a React application to other apps, such as web APIs or JavaScript frameworks, as well as for setting timers using setTimeout and setInterval.

Each component instance has 5 updating lifecycle methods, which are invoked in the following sequence whenever a component instance is modified (Figure 5.2):

1. **componentWillReceiveProps:** It is only when a component instance is set to accept props that component Will Receive Props is called prior to rendering.

2. **shouldComponentUpdate:** This accepts two parameters by default: nextProps and nextState. nextProps and nextState are often compared to this.props and this.state. If the value of shouldComponentUpdate is true, nothing occurs. If ShouldComponentUpdate, on the other hand, returns false, the component would not be updated.

3. **Render:** We've been talking about it the whole time.

4. **componentWillUpdate:** So, in between the render and shouldCompoundUpdate, componentWillUpdate is invoked. nextProps and nextState are the two parameters it gets. This isn't anything we can name. componentWillUpdate has a setState method. Its primary function is to interact with things outside the application.

5. **componentDidUpdate:** prevProps and prevState are automatically supplied to component Did Update when it is called. These are pointers to the component's pre-update properties and state, which are not updated during this time. You may see how they compare to the present props and condition of affairs by comparing them.

6. **componentWillUnmount:** When a component is about to be deleted from the DOM, this method is called.

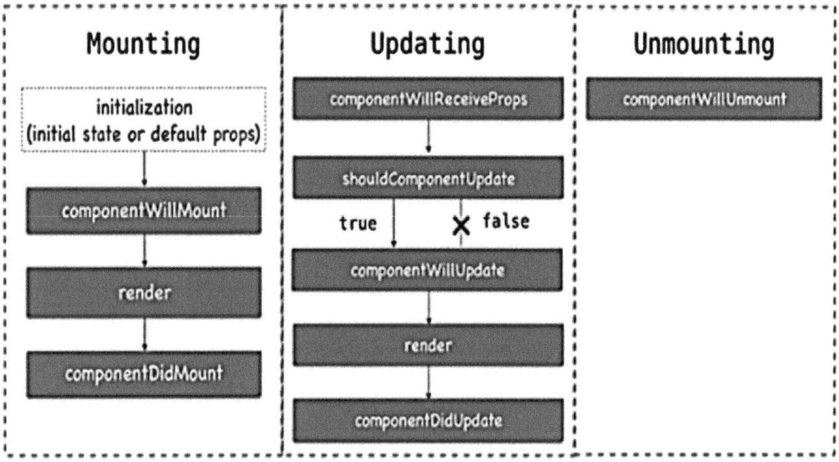

FIGURE 5.2 Lifecycle methods of ReactJS.

5.3.6 REACTJS HOOKS

React Conf 2018 saw an important innovation in the world of React, namely 'Hooks' (available from v16.8.0), which allows us to use Stateful Component features in Functional Components. Hooks are a type of functionality that allows us to integrate React state and lifecycle elements without requiring Classes, as well as structure the code within a component into reusable, independent parts.

We were constructing an app with a faster load time and enhanced user experience while overhauling our website with React and OOJs, but how did our JavaScript bundle look? Babel was converting our code to browser-friendly JS. React components created with Classes were turned into larger chunks in this transpiled code, but functional components remained smaller. This piqued my interest.

Is OOJs truly the answer to our challenge of making a quick and compact app? If it creates smaller code chunks, why not functional programming? How can we make our bundles smaller? This was the time when we discovered the freshly released React Hooks, which offered a means to create functional stateful components while also reducing bundle size. Using Hooks also improved the manageability and reusability of our business logic.

5.3.7 MOTIVATION FOR USING HOOKS

We saw the rise and fall of Functional Programming, but in the past few years, we have witnessed a steep rise in Functional Programming over OOP.

This changing trend brought our focus on functional programming making our code:

- Easier to read and test;
- Less code;
- Performance boost for the functional component.

5.4 APPLICATION PROGRAMMING INTERFACE (API)

Application Programming Interface (API) is a software middleman that enables two apps to communicate with one another. Each time you use a social media app such as Facebook, send an instant message or monitor a delivery guy on a food ordering app such as Zomato or Swiggy, you are using an application programming interface (API).

5.4.1 UNDERSTANDING APIS USING AN EXAMPLE

The above definition might have confused you a bit, but here is a detailed explanation for the same. You might have used applications such as Zomato, Swiggy, Ola, Uber, etc. Ever wondered what's common in all these applications? All of these have a map using which we get the real-time tracking of the delivery boy or driver.

Now, these apps have not developed or implemented their map, so how do they have one on their website or app? The answer to this is that they use a system called "Google Maps" which many of you might have used in the form of an app.

These apps cannot access the Google Maps system directly; instead, they interact with a security layer of Google Maps, commonly known as the Google Maps API (Figure 5.3).

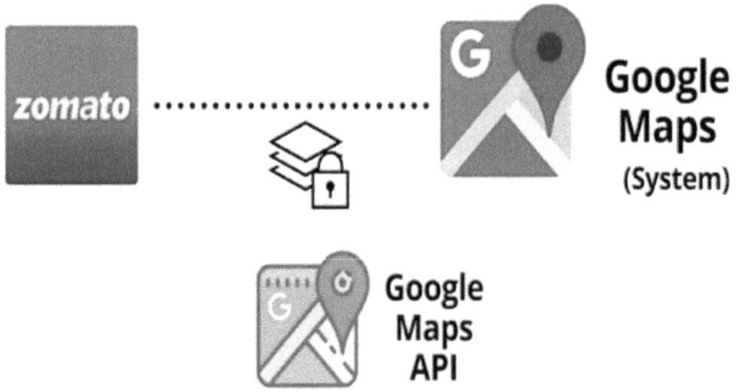

FIGURE 5.3 Zomato using Google Maps API.

So, if Zomato wants to access certain data, it won't directly ask the Google Maps system for it; rather, it will send a request to the Google Maps API. If the Google Maps system approves the API request made from Zomato, it will send the required data to Zomato using the API. And if it doesn't approve the request, it will return an "Error Message."

So, the API tells us about "What" of the system and not "How." What does it mean? If the system has a recipe for making a burger, the API won't talk about the recipe of the burger; rather, it will just take the complete burger and give it to the app/website. Thus, the API could be understood as a messenger that transfers data from one application to another, avoiding direct access between the two applications. We spoke about the API providing a "layer of security." We'll talk in detail about how the API does so. Since the server and your phone are never totally isolated from one another, your personal information is never at risk of being compromised. Instead, they link to each other through little data packets, providing just the data that is needed, like ordering takeout—instead of relying on a centralized network.

In this system, you tell a restaurant what you want to eat, and they explain what they need in return. Then you receive what you asked for.

5.5 FETCHING DATA FROM APIS

The Fetch API offers a straightforward interface for retrieving resources. When compared to the earlier XML HTTP request, which usually demands the inclusion of extra code, Fetch streamlines the process of performing online queries and managing replies. If you've ever worked with the XML Http Request (XHR) object, you'll be pleased to know that the Fetch API can accomplish all the same tasks.

Additional improvements have been made to the Fetch API, making it easier to use. To provide web browsers additional options for sending server requests, this application employs the Promise programming language. This technique instructs web browsers to make a request to a URL by using the global scope method fetch().

5.5.1 API REQUEST

The fetch() function only accepts one argument, the resource's URL:

```
let response = fetch(url);
```

There are two ways to handle the get() method's Promise – requested resource becomes accessible. At this point, the promise will become a Response object. The Response object wraps the fetched resource. The Response object includes several characteristics and methods for inspecting the response.

5.5.2 READING THE RESPONSE

If the answer is raw text, use the text() function. The text() function returns a Promise containing the complete resource's content. In fact, you'll frequently utilize async/await with the retrieve() method, as shown below.

Aside from the text() function, the Response object offers various methods to handle different types of data, such as Json(), blob(), form Data(), and array Buffer().

5.5.3 HANDLING THE STATUS CODE OF THE RESPONSE

In the Response object, both status and status Text properties describe the status. A successful request has a status code of 200 and a textual description of OK. Unable to locate requested resources will result in an HTTP error message "404 Not Found." If the requested address encounters a server error, the code will be 500.

If the requesting address gets redirected to another with a response of 300–309, the Response object's status is set to 200. True for the rerouted property as well. The promise returned by get() rejects when it encounters a genuine failure, such as an internet browser timeout, a broken network connection, or a CORS breach.

5.5.4 *EXAMPLE OF FETCH API*

Let's say you have the data shown in Figure 5.4 in a Json file on your webserver:

```
[{
        "username": "john",
        "firstName": "John",
        "lastName": "Doe",
        "gender": "Male",
        "profileURL": "img/male.png",
        "email": "john.doe@example.com"
    },
    {
        "username": "jane",
        "firstName": "Jane",
        "lastName": "Doe",
        "gender": "Female",
        "profileURL": "img/female.png",
        "email": "jane.doe@example.com"
    }
]
```

FIGURE 5.4 Inside a Json file.

Figure 5.5 shows the HTML page:

```
<!DOCTYPE html>
<html lang="en">
<head>
    <meta charset="UTF-8">
    <meta name="viewport" content="width=device-width, initial-scale=1.0">
    <title>Fetch API Demo</title>
    <link rel="stylesheet" href="css/style.css">
</head>
<body>
    <div class="container"></div>
    <script src="js/app.js"></script>
</body>
</html>
```

FIGURE 5.5 Html File.

Our app.js file will make use of the get() function in order to retrieve the users 'data and then display it inside the container classed <div> element. In order to begin, you must define the getUsers() method. The server provides Json (Figure 5.6).

```
async function getUsers() {
    let url = 'users.json';
    try {
        let res = await fetch(url);
        return await res.json();
    } catch (error) {
        console.log(error);
    }
}
```

FIGURE 5.6 Example of Fetch() method.

The render Users() method, which displays user data, should then be created (Figure 5.7):

```
async function renderUsers() {
    let users = await getUsers();
    let html = '';
    users.forEach(user => {
        let htmlSegment = `<div class="user">
                            <img src="${user.profileURL}" >
                            <h2>${user.firstName} ${user.lastName}</h2>
                            <div class="email"><a href="email:${user.email}">${user.email}</a></div>
                        </div>`;

        html += htmlSegment;
    });

    let container = document.querySelector('.container');
    container.innerHTML = html;
}

renderUsers();
```

FIGURE 5.7 Render() method.

5.6 FIREBASE

Developers may use Google's Firebase platform to build mobile and web apps. When it first began in 2011, it was a stand-alone company. In 2014, Google acquired the platform and has since made it their primary tool for developing mobile applications.

5.6.1 FEATURES

1. **Firebase Realtime Database:** User data may be stored and accessed in real-time using the Firebase real-time database.
2. **Cloud Firestore:** Powered by Firebase and Google Cloud Platform, Cloud Firestore is an extensible, scalable database for use in mobile, web, and server applications.
3. **Firebase Storage:** User-generated material, such as files and photographs, may be uploaded and stored in Firebase Storage.

4. **Cloud Functions for Firebase:** When a Firebase feature or HTTPS request triggers an event, these may immediately launch backend code.
5. **Firebase Cloud Messaging:** For free, you may use Firebase Cloud Messaging to send messages across many platforms.
6. **Firebase Performance Monitoring:** App performance problems may be tracked with the aid of Firebase Performance Monitoring.
7. **Google Analytics:** It is a free app measuring tool that gives you information about how people use your app and how engaged they are with it.
8. **Remote Config:** It is a cloud service that allows you to update your app's behavior and look without forcing users to refresh it.
9. **App Check:** Your backend resources are protected against fraud and phishing by App Check. In order to protect your data, it may be used with both Firebase and your backends. Basically, Firebase is a combination of server and database. It has Firestore for the database, and Google OAuth (login/logout feature) is provided by the server.

5.6.2 PROS AND CONS OF FIREBASE

There are several benefits of using Firebase. In addition to the benefits, there are also some drawbacks. Take a closer look at these benefits and drawbacks:

- Advantages:
  - A real-time database is Firebase;
  - It's the most sophisticated hosted BaaS solution available;
  - It is safe;
  - It has enormous storage capacity;
  - Firebase is a serverless platform;
  - It uses JSON storage, which implies that data and objects are not separated;
  - To power applications with data, no server infrastructure is necessary;

- We have easy access to data, files, authentication, and other features;
- It has a very simple setup.

➢ **Disadvantages:**

- It lacks map-reduce capabilities;
- It does not allow for aggregation;
- Its searching and indexing capabilities are severely restricted;
- Firebase for businesses isn't extensively utilized or battle-tested.

5.6.3 FIREBASE HOSTING

Google's Firebase hosting service provides customers with safe, rapid, free, and easy access to static web material.

To make your website https-secure, you'll need to pay for an SSL certificate, which is not included in most free web hosting plans. Using the Firebase service is free of charge. As a result, it will not cost you a penny. Without a separate CDN, it provides exceptional performance across a wide range of geographic locations (Figure 5.8).

1. **A Google Account:** It's possible that you already have a Google Mail (Gmail) account, in which case that will suffice. Make one if you don't already have one.

2. **Firebase-CLI:** Before you can use the Firebase CLI, you must first install Node.js on your computer.

   After you've installed NodeJs, run the following command with npm (the Node Package Manager) to install the Firebase CLI:

   ```
   npm install -g firebase-tools
   ```

3. **Web Domain:** In the world, there are a variety of domain name providers. You can also purchase one at GoDaddy.

➢ **Steps:**

- **Step I: Developing the Firebase Project:** Sign into Firebase using your Google account.

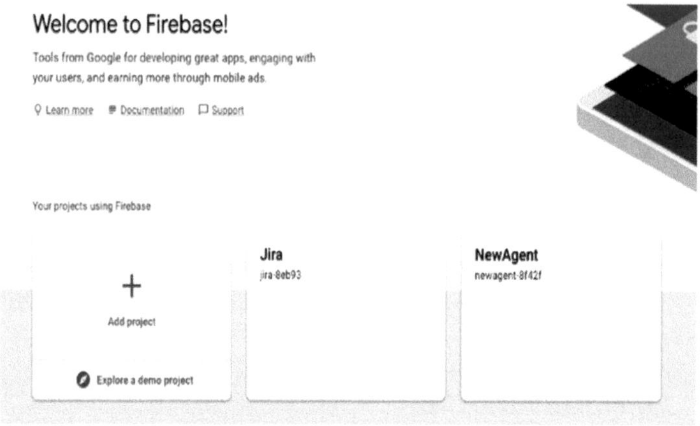

FIGURE 5.8 The landing page of Firebase.

Then create a new project and give it a name (Figure 5.9).

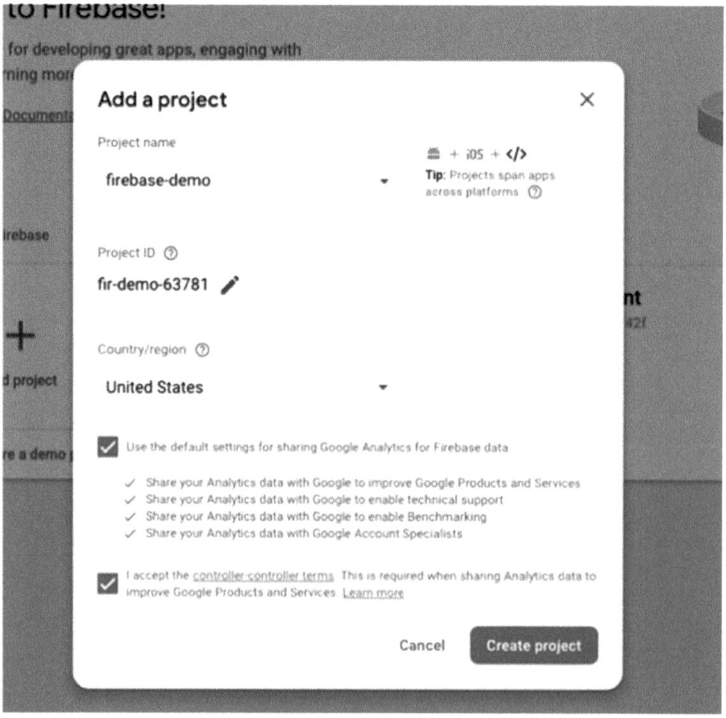

FIGURE 5.9 Creating a project in Firebase.

- **Step 2: Log in to Firebase:** Return to the command prompt and navigate to your project folder:

  cd firebase-demo

  To begin, we must use the command line to log into Firebase. Fill in the blanks with the following command:

  firebase login

  It will take you to the sign-in page in the browser.

- **Step 3: Initialize the Project:** To initiate the Firebase project, type the following command:

  firebase init

  Then select the Hosting feature and press Enter (Figure 5.10).

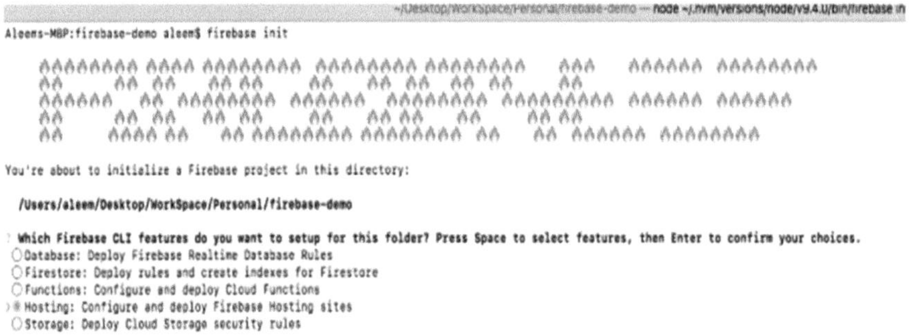

FIGURE 5.10 Firebase project initialization.

Next, select the Firebase project that we created in Step 1 when asked to do so (Figure 5.11).

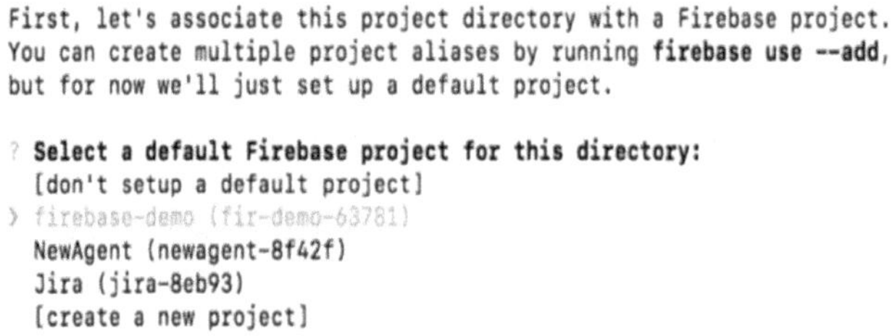

FIGURE 5.11 Select a project from Firebase.

A prompt will appear asking for the root folder of your website's assets to be entered (Figure 5.12).

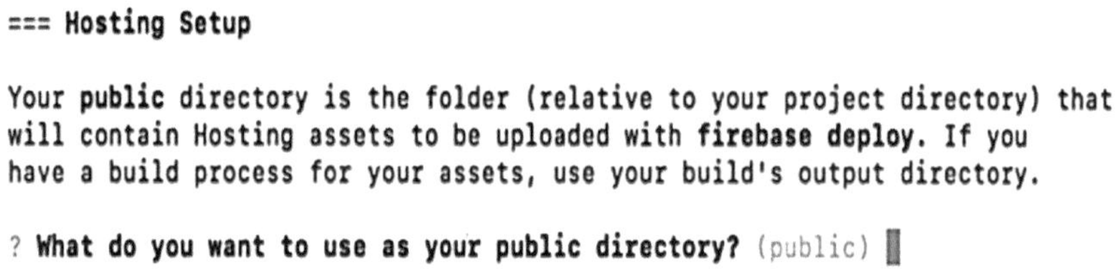

FIGURE 5.12 Entering in the main folder.

It will ask if your application is single-page or multi-page; for now, select y (Figure 5.13).

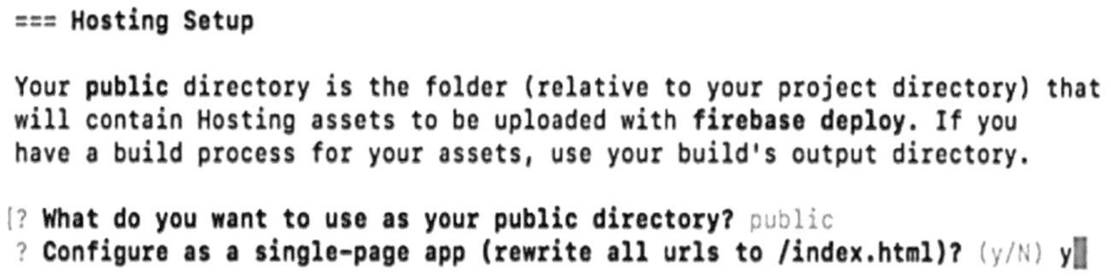

FIGURE 5.13 Single page application.

To prevent it from overriding your index.html, type n (Figure 5.14).

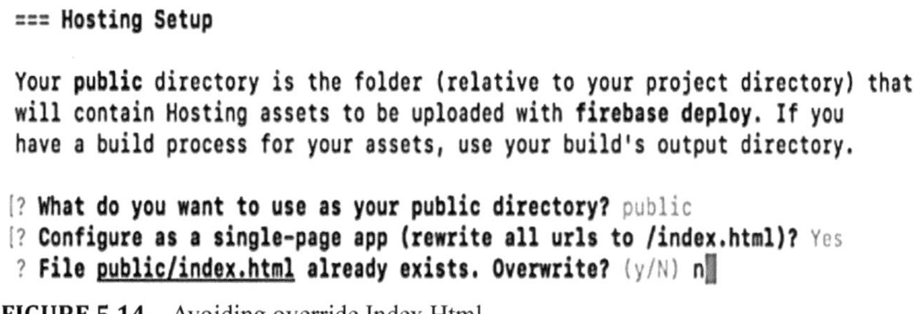

FIGURE 5.14 Avoiding override Index.Html.

- **Step 4: Verifying the Set-Up (Optional):** If everything goes well, you can run commands to check your website locally.

firebase serves

By default, it will run your website on http://localhost:5000 (Figure 5.15).

```
[Aleems-MBP:firebase-demo aleem$ firebase serve

=== Serving from '/Users/aleem/Desktop/WorkSpace/Personal/firebase-demo'...

i  hosting: Serving hosting files from: public
✔  hosting: Local server: http://localhost:5000
```

FIGURE 5.15 Check your website locally.

- **Step 5: Firebase Deployment:** You must run commands in order to deploy your project (Figure 5.16).

```
[Aleems-MBP:firebase-demo aleem$ firebase deploy

=== Deploying to 'fir-demo-63781'...

i  deploying hosting
i  hosting: preparing public directory for upload...
✔  hosting: 1 files uploaded successfully

✔  Deploy complete!

Project Console: https://console.firebase.google.com/project/fir-demo-63781/overview
Hosting URL: https://fir-demo-63781.firebaseapp.com
Aleems-MBP:firebase-demo aleem$
```

FIGURE 5.16 Final deployment of the project.

That's how simple it is to get your website up and running on Firebase.

5.7 METHODOLOGY

During the software's creation, several procedures were taken to reflect the coronavirus data as accurately as feasible. As a result, the exact data is presented to users in a variety of formats, including graphical and geographic representations.

The following are the steps taken during the creation of this project:

1. The basic structure of the application was created before the implementation of any code. The structure was designed in such a way that the whole UI looks like a single web page and there are not too many instructions for the user to reach a particular data.

2. The coding phase of the website was initiated and planned in such a way that when a particular variable changes, the component in the DOM associated with it automatically changes. For example: Map Automatically Changes as You Search (Figure 5.17).

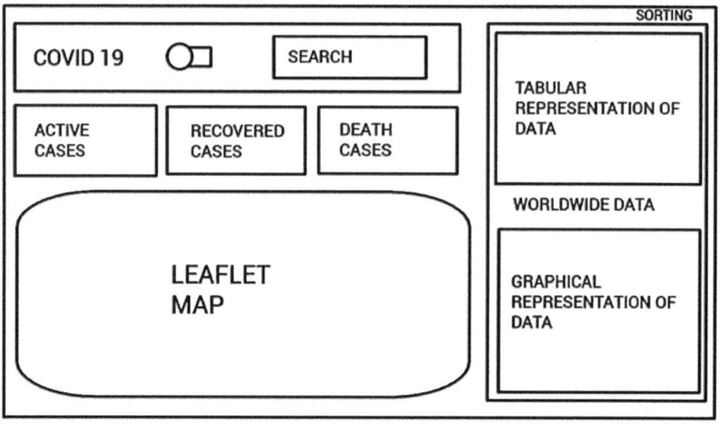

FIGURE 5.17 The basic structure of the application.

3. The coding was performed in a hierarchical manner such that the parent component was implemented first, and then the child components were implemented. For example, Parent Component: App Child Componcnt.
4. As the app was coded with components, it made the code reusable.
5. An API call was made to disease.sh in order to get data. GET requests were made to endpoints provided by disease.sh.
6. All data fetching calls were made using React JS's use Effect() hook, which takes two parameters: an async function that describes what to do and a second argument that specifies when to run that function.
7. After collecting the data, it was transformed into the required formats, as the required format for graphs is X, Coordinates.
8. CSS and Material UI were also used as a helping hand to make this website much more attractive.
9. Two modes of web view are also provided for convenience: the user dark mode and light mode.
10. An API call was made to disease.sh to get data. GET requests were made to endpoints provided by disease.sh.

11. React's use Effect() hook takes two parameters: an async function describing what to do and a second argument specifying when to run the function. All data-fetching calls were made under this hook.
12. After collecting the data, it was transformed to the required formats as the required format for graphs is X, Coordinates.
13. CSS and Material UI are also used as a helping hand to make this website much more attractive.
14. Two modes of web view are also provided for convenience: the user dark mode and light mode (Figure 5.18).

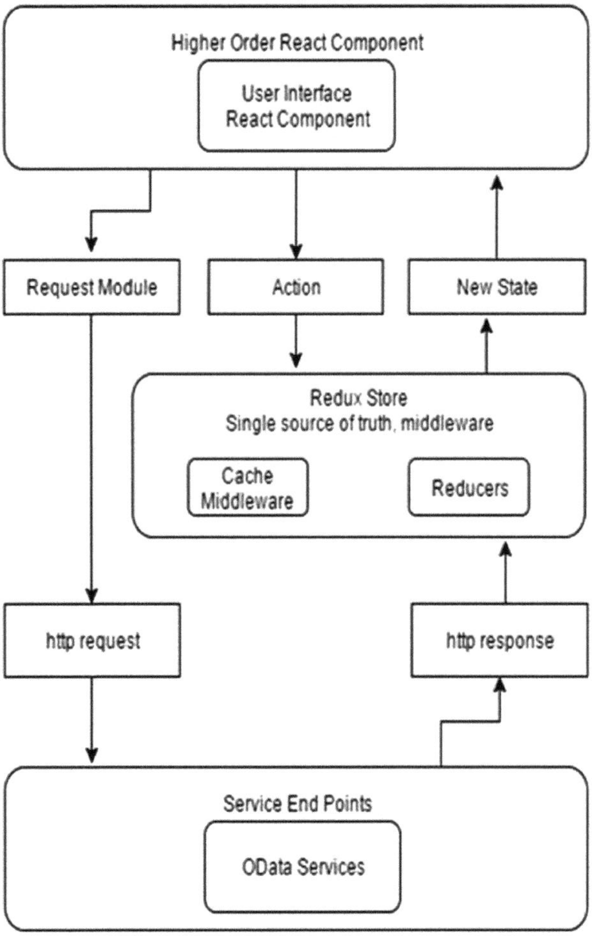

FIGURE 5.18 Architecture of ReactJS applications.

Precise data representation and data modification are the main aims behind a website that serves figures related to any pandemic or healthcare issue [8].

5.8 RESULT

The completed web application is an excellent example of software that incorporates all of React JS's features and provides the best user interface for users [5]. In both dark and bright conditions, the data representation is accurate and well-managed, and the color combinations used in the project are well-managed. This will allow a user from anywhere in the world to look at global data or search for specific countries and data kinds. All these characteristics contribute to the responsive and beautiful user interface [4] of this online application, making it simple to use (Figure 5.19).

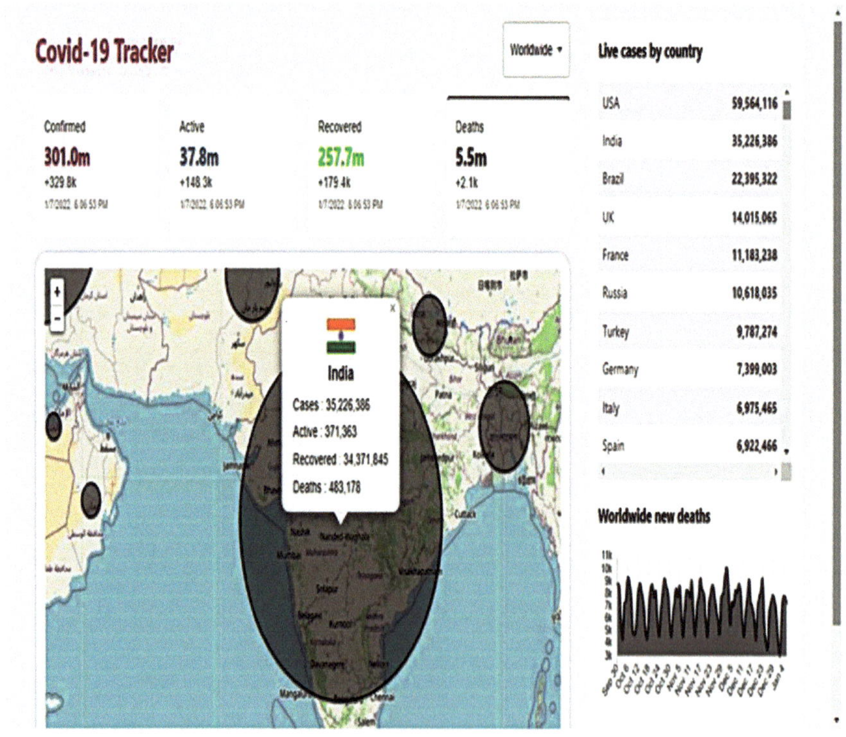

FIGURE 5.19 Corona tracker project snapshot.

5.9 FUTURE SCOPE AND CONCLUSION

More intriguing features, such as disease prediction based on symptoms and guidance for the next steps, such as finding a suitable doctor in the user's area, will greatly enhance this program.

These will aid in the study and development of new algorithms for locating doctors in a user's neighborhood. This is a burgeoning research field that is still ongoing for real-time observation of enormous crowds. We may deduce from this application that ReactJS and some basic front-end development techniques can lead to such an engaging web application with a variety of capabilities. Though the program is now somewhat simple, it has a lot of room for sophisticated topics and technologies to be added in the future, and for the time being, it is accomplishing the goal for which it was created.

KEYWORDS

- **corona tracker**
- **firebase project**
- **monitoring COVID-19**
- **ReactJS**
- **status code**
- **web application**

REFERENCES

1. Lu, R., Zhao, X., Li, J., Niu, P., Yang, B., Wu, H., et al. (2020). Genomic characterization and epidemiology of 2019 novel coronavirus: implications for virus origins and receptor binding. *The Lancet*, *395*(10224), 565–574.
2. Carroll, L. N., Au, A. P., Detwiler, L. T., Fu, T. C., Painter, I. S., & Abernethy, N. F. (2014). Visualization and analytics tools for infectious disease epidemiology: a systematic review. *Journal of Biomedical Informatics, 51*, 287–298.
3. Valls, J., Tobias, A., Satorra, P., & Tebe, C. (2020). COVID-19-tracker: a shiny app to analyze data on SARS-CoV-2 epidemic in Spain. *Gaceta Sanitaria, 35*, 99–101. https://doi.org/10.1016/j.gaceta.2020.04.002.

4. Dong, E., Du, H., & Gardner, L. (2020). An interactive web-based dashboard to track COVID-19 in real time. *The Lancet Infectious Diseases, 20*(5), 533–534.
5. Wolkewitz, M., & Puljak, L. (2020). Methodological challenges of analyzing COVID-19 data during the pandemic. *BMC Medical Research Methodology, 20*(1), 81.
6. Lauer, S. A., Grantz, K. H., Bi, Q., Jones, F. K., Zheng, Q., Meredith, H. R., et al. (2020). The incubation period of coronavirus disease 2019 (COVID-19) from publicly reported confirmed cases: estimation and application. *Annals of Internal Medicine, 172*(9), 577–582.
7. Roser, M., Ritchie, H., Ortiz-Ospina, E., & Hasell, J. (2020). Coronavirus pandemic (COVID-19). Published online at OurWorldInData.org. *University of Oxford.*
8. Kaur, D. N., Sahdev, S. L., Chaturvedi, V., & Rajawat, D. (2020). Fighting COVID-19 with technology and innovation, evolving and advancing with technological possibilities. International *Journal of Advanced Research in Engineering and Technology (IJARET, 11*(7), 395–405.

CHAPTER 6

Investigation of Diagnosing Irregularities in Endodontic Applications Using Deep Learning Methods

A. AISHWARIYA,[1] K. A. SUNITHA,[2] and K. T. MAGESH[3]

[1]*Department of Electronics and Instrumentation Engineering, SRM Institute of Science and Technology, Chennai, Tamil Nadu, India*

[2]*Department of Electronics and Communication Engineering, SRM University, Andhra Pradesh, India*

[3]*Department of Oral Pathology and Microbiology, SRM Kattankulathur Dental College and Hospital, Tamil Nadu, India*

ABSTRACT

In dentistry, endodontics is the study of dental pulp and tissues surrounding the roots. Endodontic treatment is otherwise called root canal treatment. The importance of endodontics focuses on several therapies to protect human teeth from cavities or infections, injuries, and various oral diseases like oral cancer and periodontal disease. Over 3.5 billion people are affected by various oral diseases, 10% of the global population is affected by periodontal diseases, and 530 million children suffer from tooth decay. There are different types of root canal morphology and configurations in which multiple abnormalities exist, such as C-shaped canals, fusion of roots, dens invaginatus, distolingual root, taurodontism, root dilaceration, etc. AI plays a vital role in endodontic applications. Using AI for the

Data-Driven Analytics for Healthcare: Artificial Intelligence and Machine Learning for Medical Diagnostics. Meghna Sharma, Priyanka Vashisht, A. V. Senthil Kumar, Chitra Singh, and Abdelmalek Amine (Eds.)

prediction and diagnosis of periapical lesions, root fractures can be detected. Nowadays, AI is used to determine working length measurements, predict dental pulp stem cells, and guide retreatment procedures. Therefore, AI provides successful outcomes and improvements in diagnosis and prediction in root canal applications in day-to-day practices. This review chapter summarizes different deep learning techniques that can be implemented in various endodontic applications in detail to understand the pros and cons.

6.1 INTRODUCTION

Endodontics is the study of dental pulp and tissues surrounding the roots. The term "endo" means "inside" and "odont" means "tooth." Endodontic treatment is otherwise called root canal treatment. Endodontic treatment aims to preserve and restore the pulp by properly cleaning, shaping, and filling the roots of the tooth. Therefore, endodontics is used for the diagnosis of dental pulp and periapical tissue diseases. The periapical tissues are unique when compared to the oral tissues since these tissues are minute or invisible to the endodontist. The goal of endodontic treatment is to restore and save the tooth from infections and decay. Different types of tests are performed before endodontic treatment, including palpation, percussion, periodontal probing, thermal testing, and pulp testing.

6.2 STATISTICS OF ENDODONTICS TREATMENTS

Oral diseases are widespread diseases globally and have a greater impact on general health and economic status of the people [1]. The Global Burden of Disease found that oral conditions remain a substantial population health challenge. Around 3.5 billion cases of oral conditions, of which 2.3 billion are untreated tooth infections in permanent teeth, 532 million had untreated decay in deciduous teeth, 796 million are severely affected by periodontitis disease, 267 million had tooth loss, and 139 million had other oral conditions [2]. Figures 6.1(a) and 6.1(b) represent the age (10 to 83) group population undergoing root canal treatment, as a result 47.19% suffer from root canal treatment at the age group of 21 to 41 years and 36.40% of molar teeth undergo more frequent diagnostic tests since they are more prone to dental caries [3].

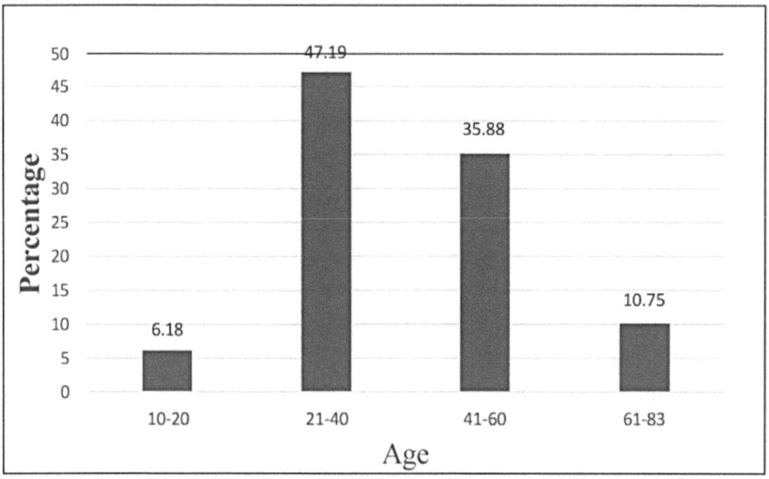

FIGURE 6.1(A) Graphs represents the age groups of the population undergo root canal.

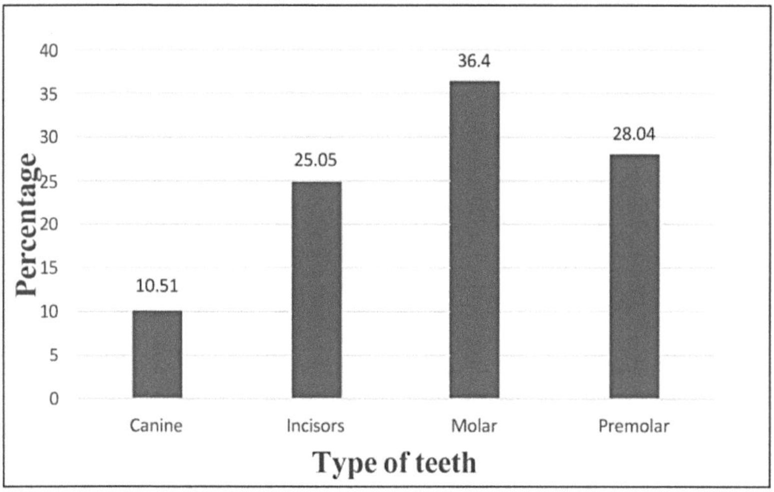

FIGURE 6.1(B) Graph represents different type of teeth undergone root canal.

6.3 APPLICATION AND IMPORTANCE OF ENDODONTICS

The main aim of endodontics is to eliminate or reduce bacterial infections using endodontic instruments for cleaning and tooth filling to save the tooth from decay. It is also used to restore the pulpal tissues from inflammations [4].

6.3.1 ELECTRONIC AND DIGITAL TECHNOLOGIES IN ENDODONTIC TREATMENT

In digital dentistry, applications in endodontics play a vital role. Digital applications, such as digital two-dimensional (2D) imaging and three-dimensional (3D) imaging techniques, computer-aided diagnosis (CAD) and artificial intelligence (AI) models, computer-controlled access cavity designs, and 3D printing applications, etc., are advancing. The advancement in digital dentistry applications, especially for visualization techniques for root canal anatomy like two-dimensional (2D) and three-dimensional (3D) radiography and Cone-beam computed tomography (CBCT), are used. The major objective of endodontics is to eliminate bacteria present in the roots of the tooth. It is also used to eradicate inflammations in pulpal tissue [4].

Therefore, digital technologies provide useful information for the diagnosis and treatment of endodontic applications. The digital technologies include Conventional pulp testing, Laser Doppler flowmetry, Pulse oximetry, Allodynia measuring device, Optical coherence tomography (OCT), and digital radiographs such as CBCT, MRI, ultrasound.

Electronic technologies used in endodontics include microscopes and endoscopes for magnification purposes, Sonic and ultrasonic devices, electronic apex locator used for the working length determination in root canal treatments [6].

6.4 ROLE OF IMAGING IN ENDODONTICS

Imaging in endodontics application takes place in three different stages [7]:

1. **Preoperative Stage:** During the preoperative stage, the imaging techniques help to analyze the morphology of dental and alveolar hard tissue, especially in pathological alterations of teeth. This includes the location of the root canal, the number of roots and their structure, the direction and curvature of roots, pulp chamber size, calcifications of the tooth. It is also used to diagnose root fractures and crown issues.

2. **Intraoperative Stage:** In this stage, imaging techniques help determine the working length of the root canal and analyze the changes that occur in the tooth and bone.

3. **Postoperative Stage:** During this stage, imaging techniques help evaluate the filling and sealing of the tooth with root canal materials and find any changes that occur in the tooth and periapical hard tissue after treatment, as well as any surgical considerations.

6.5 IRREGULARITIES IN ENDODONTIC TREATMENTS

Root canal treatment has a high success rate, even though it is a difficult, invasive, and complex procedure. Complications during root canal procedures can occur due to a lack of understanding of the structure and iatrogenic errors during instrumentation. Some problems can be solved, while others cannot be predicted. Due to these irregularities, retreatment may be required either through surgical or nonsurgical methods. Irregularities include reinfection, missed root canals, crown fractures, fractured instruments, postoperative pain, and post-treatment issues.

6.5.1 REINFECTION

Due to poor cleaning, shaping, obturation, or sealing procedures, poor restorations, and fractures are a few problems that make root canal treatment failure. The major short-term cause of root canal treatment failure is "reinfection" or "persistent infection" [11].

6.5.2 MISSED ROOT CANAL

The canal structures can vary and be complex. When the patient has a complex tooth structure, there is a chance of clinicians missing the canal. Therefore, 3D radiographic imaging like CBCT can be used to reduce such errors [12].

6.5.3 CROWN FRACTURES

Crown or root fractures can be detected in the preoperative, intraoperative, and postoperative stages of root canal treatment. The major cause of long-term root canal failures is root fracture [13]. Depending on the severity of the fracture, the endodontist decides whether tooth extraction or filling is required.

6.5.4 FRACTURED INSTRUMENTS

When the canal structure is complex and curved, instruments undergo more stress than the mechanical resistance of the instrument. This results in failure and affects the shaping and cleaning procedures in root canal treatment. Therefore, endodontists should be more careful in handling instruments to avoid overstressing them [14, 15].

6.5.5 POSTOPERATIVE PAIN AND POST-TREATMENT

This postoperative pain occurs after root canal procedures and should be addressed immediately [16]. If the tooth remains symptomatic after a month or a year, it is a sign of treatment failure. Symptoms may include pain when chewing, inflammation, etc. Sometimes complications arise after dental treatments, requiring further endodontic treatment [17].

6.6 LITERATURE REVIEW ON CLINICAL DIAGNOSTIC TOOLS FOR ENDODONTIC APPLICATIONS

Various digital clinical applications are used in endodontics, such as digital two-dimensional (2D) and three-dimensional (3D) imaging techniques, computer-aided diagnosis (CAD) and artificial intelligence (AI) models, computer-controlled access cavity designs, and 3D printing applications [18] (Table 6.1).

6.7 ROLE OF ARTIFICIAL INTELLIGENCE (AI) IN ENDODONTICS AND ITS APPLICATION

Artificial Intelligence (AI) plays a vital role in dentistry. AI has the capability to mimic human intelligence and is used to perform complex decision-making, prediction, diagnosis, and treatment in healthcare applications. Nowadays, AI has increased its presence in various applications in dentistry, particularly in endodontics.

There are two types of AI present in the healthcare domain: virtual and physical [31]. The virtual type uses mathematical model algorithms for diagnosis and prediction [32], imaging techniques [33], and electronic health records. The physical type includes robots in surgery [34].

TABLE 6.1 Types of Imaging Modalities Used in Endodontics

Imaging Modalities	Principle and Application	Advantage	Disadvantage	References
Ultrasound imaging	US images can be used to view normal and diseased bones and soft tissues of the oral regions.	Portability ionizing radiation low-cost availability and accessibility.	Limited imaging depth. Image resolution is less.	[7, 19, 21]
Computed tomography (CT) imaging	CT images helps to view the soft tissues, bone, and vessels. The application like identification of anatomical structures, chronic apical periodontitis, vertical root fracture, diagnosis of multiple root canals.	High accuracy and resolution and scan time reduction.	Higher radiation expensive.	[22–24]
Magnetic resonance imaging (MRI) imaging	MRI imaging is used to study the skeletal physiology, tumors, and healings. It has the high contrast resolution in medical imaging techniques. It also used to examine inflammations and scar tissues.	Reliability portable real-time imaging.	Limited accuracy specificity and sensitivity.	[25, 26]
Infrared thermography imaging	Thermography imaging is used to evaluate the temperature changes inside the oral cavity, evaluate the thermal effects during the filling, detects the inflammation due to periodontal disease or diseases of the temporomandibular joint.	High accuracy and resolution and scan time reduction.	Limited accuracy specificity and sensitivity.	[27–29]
THz spectroscopy imaging	Terahertz imaging can play a major role in dentistry Terahertz pulsed imaging (TPI) can be utilized in the early detection of dental caries and defects in the tooth structure, Enamel erosion and diagnosis of dental pulp vitality.	Reliability portable real-time imaging.	Low speed, complicated operation.	[30]

AI techniques or algorithms learn important features using standard algorithms like random forest (RF), support vector machine (SVM), artificial neural networks (ANNs), etc., which resemble biological neurons. In deep learning, multiple layers of neurons are used to generate billions of neural connection weights that are changed and enable learning of nonlinear correlations of features [35].

6.7.1 ARTIFICIAL INTELLIGENCE (AI) IN ENDODONTICS

6.7.1.1 DETECTION

Using AI prediction and diagnosis of periapical lesions, root fractures can be detected. Nowadays AI is used to work on the working of the root canal, the capability of predicting the stem cells of dental pulp, and retreatment procedures. Therefore, AI provides successful outcomes and improvement in diagnosis and prediction in root canal applications in day-to-day practices (Table 6.2).

1. **Periapical Lesions Detection:** The diagnosis of periapical lesions is a very challenging task for endodontists. Around 75% of inflammatory lesions are due to a disease called apical periodontitis [36]. Therefore, early diagnosis will increase the success rate of treatment [37], avoid spreading to surrounding tissues, and reduce further complications.

   `The radiographs of apical periodontitis provide a compressed 2D image of a 3D object. Hence, the information from the radiographs is not accurate [38]. Cone-beam computed tomography (CBCT) imaging technique is used to detect the periapical lesion, with respect to its size and location.

   A meta-analysis reports an accuracy of 0.96 for CBCT imaging, 0.73 for conventional periapical radiograph images, and 0.72 for digital periapical radiograph images in detecting periapical lesions [39]. However, diagnosing apical periodontitis shows less accuracy, especially in root-filled teeth [40].

2. **Detection of Root Fractures:** Around 2%–5% of crown fractures are vertical root fractures (VRFs), and this leads to either resection of roots or tooth extraction [41, 42]. VRFs are detected

using radiographs and CBCT imaging techniques, and it is also very difficult to diagnose. Due to the poor diagnosis, unnecessary surgery or tooth extraction may be required. CBCT imaging is better than radiography in the case of unfilled teeth with VRFs, whereas radiographs are only slightly better for root-filled teeth than CBCT [43].

The detection of VRFs using CNN values results in a sensitivity of 0.75, precision of 0.93, and an F score of 0.83 [44]. Therefore, crown fracture detection using CBCT images yields better results, such as accuracy, when compared with radiographic images [45].

3. **Working Length Determination:** The very important step in endodontic treatment is the working length determination. Multiple methods are used for working length determination. The methods are radiography, the patient's response to a file inserted in the root canal, electronic apex locators, CBCT imaging, and digital tactile sense [46–49]. Radiography and electronic apex locators are commonly used for the working length determination by clinicians.

   Digital radiography plays a vital role because of the quality of the images in the precise interpretation of root canal morphology [50]. But still, other factors affect radiographs which result in poor detection [51]. Therefore, computer-based methods are used for the determination of accurate working lengths in endodontics.

   ANN provides high accuracy in the determination of the working length of root canal treatment [52]. ANN performs with 96% accuracy, higher than the endodontist's 76% in minor anatomic constriction determination using periapical radiographic images. Therefore, ANN can be considered an accurate method for the determination of working length.

4. **Morphology of Root and Root Canal:** CBCT and periapical radiographs are more commonly used imaging techniques in root morphology. Understanding the variation in root and root canal structure is very important for the success of nonsurgical endodontic treatment. CBCT imaging has high accuracy in imaging the root and canal compared to radiographic imaging.

Deep learning methods result in high levels of accuracy, especially in diagnosing single and multiple root structures [53]. Therefore, AI has the capability to measure the curvatures of the root canal [54].

5. **Prediction of Retreatment:** A case study or survey is used to predict the need for nonoperative root canal retreatment. The case study involves providing solutions to previous similar problems [55]. This helps in determining whether retreatment is necessary or not. It also includes data information such as recall values, performance, and probability statistics. The only limitation is that the prediction result will be as good as the information present in the data [56].

TABLE 6.2 AI Applications in Endodontics

Application	AI Techniques	Results	References
Periapical lesions detection.	Machine learning, convolution neural network, deep learning.	Radiograph and CBCT images the periapical lesions are detected. By using AI accuracy of detection is improved and that helps the clinicians to diagnose. Accuracy = 0.96 3D imaging and 0.73 (conventional periapical radiograph) and 0.72 (digital periapical radiography).	[39, 57]
Root fractures	Machine learning, convolution neural network.	AI is used in the detection of crown fractures and results a high accuracy. Research in the detection of the root fracture is promising and ongoing. Sensitivity of 0.75, precision of 0.93 and F score of 0.83.	[20, 42]
Determination of working length	Machine learning, artificial neural network.	ANN results 96% accuracy higher than the endodontist accuracy of 76%.	[43]
Root canal morphology	Machine learning, convolution neural network, deep learning.	Using AI algorithms curvature and the dimensions of the canal can be measured after the use of instrumentation procedure.	[49]
Prediction of retreatment	Machine learning	Different methods helps in the prediction of statistical probabilities for extraction of tooth.	[5]

6.8 CONCLUSION

The inadequate information and morphological changes of the root canal result in instrumentation errors and failure of the root canal treatment. The advancement in diagnostic tools and testing results in successful treatment and also using digital and electronic applications in endodontics helps to minimize the treatment time, reduce iatrogenic errors, and reduce pain. Advancement in endodontics results in successful treatment in dentistry. The advancement includes the type of material used, instrument or equipment, techniques, etc. Imaging in endodontics includes both digital and analog imaging techniques. Therefore, AI models provide successful outcomes and improvement in diagnosis and prediction in root canal applications.

KEYWORDS

- **C-shaped canals**
- **deep learning**
- **dens invaginatus**
- **endodontic applications**
- **fusion of roots**
- **root dilaceration**
- **taurodontism**

REFERENCES

1. Jakovljevic, A., Nikolic, N., Jacimovic, J., Pavlovic, O., Milicic, B., Beljic-Ivanovic, K., Miletic, M., Andric, M., & Milasin, J. (2020). Prevalence of apical periodontitis and conventional nonsurgical root canal treatment in general adult population: An updated systematic review and meta-analysis of cross-sectional studies published between 2012–2020. *Journal of Endodontics, 46*(10), 1371–1386. Advance online publication. https://doi.org/10.1016/j.joen.2020.07.007.
2. Vukovic, A., Warouw, T. S. S., Zaidi, Z., Zhang, Z. J., & Kassebaum, N. J. (2020). Global, regional, and national levels and trends in burden of oral conditions from 1990 to 2017: A systematic analysis for the Global Burden of Disease 2017 Study.

Journal of Dental Research, 99(4), 362–373. Advance online publication. https://doi.org/10.1177/0022034520908533.

3. Antony, M., Sugumaran, S., & Leelavathi, L. (2020). Association of diagnostic test and type of response in a single visit root canal treatment. *Journal of Research in Medical and Dental Science, 8*(7), 78–83.
4. de Carvalho Felippini, A. L. (2019). Introductory Chapter: Some important aspects of root canal treatment. In P. n. L. De Carvalho Felippini (Ed.), *Root Canal [Working Title]*. 1–8, IntechOpen. https://doi.org/10.5772/intechopen.83653.
5. Leite, A. F., van Gerven, A., Willems, H., et al. (2021). Artificial intelligence-driven novel tool for tooth detection and segmentation on panoramic radiographs. *Clinical Oral Investigations, 25*, 2257–2267.
6. Masri, R., & Driscoll, C. F. (2015). Digital applications in endodontics. In *Clinical Applications of Digital Dental Technology* (pp. 177–192). https://doi.org/10.1002/9781119045564.ch9.
7. Deepak, B. S., Narmatha, V. J., Snehil, T. K., Subash, T. S., Anamika, T., & Nandini, D. B. (2012). Imaging techniques in endodontics: An overview. *Journal of Clinical Imaging Science, 2*(1), 13. https://doi.org/10.4103/2156-7514.94227.
8. Bergenholtz, G. (2016). Assessment of treatment failure in endodontic therapy. *Journal of Oral Rehabilitation, 43*(10), 753–758. https://doi.org/10.1111/joor.12423.
9. Plotino, G., Grande, N. M., Mazza, C., et al. (2010). Influence of size and taper of artificial canals on the trajectory of NiTi rotary instruments in cyclic fatigue studies. *Oral Surgery, Oral Medicine, Oral Pathology, Oral Radiology, and Endodontology, 109*(1), e60–e66. https://doi.org/10.1016/j.tripleo.2009.08.009.
10. Gambarini, G., Seracchiani, M., Piasecki, L., et al. (2019). Measurement of torque generated during intracanal instrumentation in vivo. *International Endodontic Journal, 52*(5), 737–745. https://doi.org/10.1111/iej.13042.
11. Alghamdi, F., Alhaddad, A. J., & Abuzinadah, S. (2020). Healing of periapical lesions after surgical endodontic retreatment: A systematic review. *Cureus, 12*(2), e6916. https://doi.org/10.7759/cureus.6916.
12. Prada, I., Mico-Munoz, P., Giner-Lluesma, T., et al. (2019). Influence of microbiology on endodontic failure: Literature review. *Medicina Oral, Patologia Oral y Cirugia Bucal, 24*(3), e364–e372. https://doi.org/10.4317/medoral.22907.
13. Gambarini, G., Piasecki, L., Miccoli, G., et al. (2018). Cone-beam computed tomography in the assessment of periapical lesions in endodontically treated teeth. *European Journal of Dentistry, 12*(1), 136–143. https://doi.org/10.4103/ejd.ejd_320_17.
14. Figueiredo, F. E., Martins-Filho, P. R., & Faria-E-Silva, A. L. (2015). Do metal post-retained restorations result in more root fractures than fiber post-retained restorations? A systematic review and meta-analysis. *Journal of Endodontics, 41*(3), 309–316. https://doi.org/10.1016/j.joen.2014.10.006.
15. Gambarini, G., Piasecki, L., Miccoli, G., et al. (2019). Classification and cyclic fatigue evaluation of new kinematics for endodontic instruments. *Australian Endodontic Journal, 45*(2), 154–162. https://doi.org/10.1111/aej.12294.
16. Gambarini, G., Miccoli, G., Seracchiani, M., et al. (2018). Fatigue resistance of new and used nickel-titanium rotary instruments: A comparative study. *Clinica Terapeutica, 169*(3), e96–e101. https://doi.org/10.7417/T.2018.2061.

17. Gambarini, G., Di Nardo, D., Miccoli, G., et al. (2017). The influence of a new clinical motion for endodontic instruments on the incidence of postoperative pain. *Clinica Terapeutica, 168*(1), e23–e27. https://doi.org/10.7417/CT.2017.1977.
18. Guarnieri, R., Di Nardo, D., Gaimari, G., et al. (2019). Short vs. standard laser-microgrooved implants supporting single and splinted crowns: A prospective study with 3 years follow-up. *Journal of Prosthodontics, 28*(2), 771–779. https://doi.org/10.1111/jopr.12959.
19. Keskin, C. (2021). Digital applications in endodontics: An update and review. *Journal of Experimental and Clinical Medicine, 38*(S2), 168–174. https://doi.org/10.52142/omujecm.38.si.dent.15.
20. Ekert, T., Krois, J., Meinhold, L., et al. (2019). Deep learning for the radiographic detection of apical lesions. *Journal of Endodontics, 45*, 917–922.e5.
21. Maity, I., Kumara, A., Shukla, A. K., Usha, H. L., & Naveen, D. N. (2011). Monitoring of healing by ultrasound with color power Doppler after root canal treatment of maxillary anterior teeth with periapical lesions. *Journal of Conservative Dentistry, 14*, 252–257.
22. Yoshioka, T., Kobayashi, C., Suda, H., & Sasak, T. (2002). An observation of the healing process of periapical lesions by digital subtraction radiography. *Journal of Endodontics, 28*, 589–591.
23. Mikrogeorgis, G., Lyroudia, K., Molyvdas, I., Nikolaidis, N., & Pitas, I. (2004). Digital radiograph registration and subtraction: A useful tool for the evaluation of the progress of chronic apical periodontitis. *Journal of Endodontics, 30*, 513–516.
24. Tachibana, H., & Matsumoto, K. (1990). Applicability of X-ray computerized tomography in endodontics. *Dental Traumatology, 6*, 16–20.
25. Youssefzadeh, S., Gahleitner, A., Dorffner, R., Bernhart, T., & Kainberger, F. M. (1999). Dental vertical root fractures: Value of CT in detection. *Radiology, 21*, 545–549.
26. Nance, R., Tyndall, D., Levin, L. G., & Trope, M. (2000). Identification of root canals in molars by tuned-aperture computed tomography. *International Endodontic Journal, 33*, 392–396.
27. van Dijke, C. F., Kirk, B. A., Peterfy, C. G., Genant, H. K., Brasch, R. C., & Kapila, S. (1997). Arthritic temporomandibular joint: Correlation of macromolecular contrast-enhanced MR imaging parameters and histopathologic findings. *Radiology, 204*, 825–832.
28. Robb, R. A. (1982). The dynamic spatial reconstructor: An X-ray video-fluoroscopic CT scanner for dynamic volume imaging of moving organs. *IEEE Transactions on Medical Imaging, 1*, 22–33.
29. Kasprzyk-Kucewicz, T., Cholewka, A., Bałamut, K., Kownacki, P., Kaszuba, N., Kaszuba, M., Stanek, A., Sieroń, K., Stransky, J., Pasz, A., & Morawiec, T. (2021). The applications of infrared thermography in surgical removal of retained teeth effects assessment. *Journal of Thermal Analysis and Calorimetry, 144*, 139–144. https://doi.org/10.1007/s10973-020-09457-6.
30. Boushady, M. A., Talaat, W., Hamdoon, Z., et al. (2021). Thermography as a non-ionizing quantitative tool for diagnosing periapical inflammatory lesions. *BMC Oral Health, 21*, 260. https://doi.org/10.1186/s12903-021-01618-9.

31. Nasution, A. I., & Pankov, M. N. (2020). The advantage and basic approach of infrared thermography in dentistry. *Journal of International Dental and Medical Research, 13*(2), 731–737.
32. Hirmer, M., Danilov, S. N., Giglberger, S., Putzger, J., Niklas, A., Jäger, A., Hiller, K. A., Löffler, S., Schmalz, G., Redlich, B., Schulz, I., Monkman, G., & Ganichev, S. D. (2012). Spectroscopic study of human teeth and blood from visible to terahertz frequencies for clinical diagnosis of dental pulp vitality. *Journal of Infrared, Millimeter, and Terahertz Waves, 33*(3), 366–375. https://doi.org/10.1007/s10762-012-9872-3.
33. Hamet, P., & Tremblay, J. (2017). Artificial intelligence in medicine. *Metabolism, 69*(S), S36–S40.
34. Huang, S., Yang, J., Fong, S., & Zhao, Q. (2020). Artificial intelligence in cancer diagnosis and prognosis: Opportunities and challenges. *Cancer Letters, 471*, 61–71.
35. Gao, L., Jiao, T., Feng, Q., & Wang, W. (2021). Application of artificial intelligence in diagnosis of osteoporosis using medical images: A systematic review and meta-analysis. *Osteoporosis International, 32*, 1279–1286.
36. LeCun, Y., Bengio, Y., & Hinton, G. (2015). Deep learning. *Nature, 521*, 436–444.
37. Bhandari, M., Zeffiro, T., & Reddiboina, M. (2020). Artificial intelligence and robotic surgery: Current perspective and future directions. *Current Opinion in Urology, 30*, 48–54.
38. Becconsall-Ryan, K., Tong, D., & Love, R. M. (2010). Radiolucent inflammatory jaw lesion: A twenty-year analysis. *International Endodontic Journal, 43*, 859–865.
39. Setzer, F. C., Shi, K. J., Zhang, Z., et al. (2020). Artificial intelligence for the computer-aided detection of periapical lesions in cone-beam computed tomographic images. *Journal of Endodontics, 46*, 987–993.
40. Patel, S., Dawood, A., Whaites, E., & Pitt Ford, T. (2009). New dimensions in endodontic imaging: Part 1. Conventional and alternative radiographic systems. *International Endodontic Journal, 42*, 447–462.
41. Leonardi Dutra, K., Haas, L., Porporatti, A. L., et al. (2016). Diagnostic accuracy of cone-beam computed tomography and conventional radiography on apical periodontitis: A systematic review and meta-analysis. *Journal of Endodontics, 42*, 356–364.
42. Fuss, Z., Lustig, J., Katz, A., & Tamse, A. (2001). An evaluation of endodontically treated vertical root fractured teeth: Impact of operative procedures. *Journal of Endodontics, 27*, 46–48.
43. Talwar, S., Utneja, S., Nawal, R. R., et al. (2016). Role of cone-beam computed tomography in diagnosis of vertical root fractures: A systematic review and meta-analysis. *Journal of Endodontics, 42*, 12–24.
44. Fukuda, M., Inamoto, K., Shibata, N., et al. (2020). Evaluation of an artificial intelligence system for detecting vertical root fracture on panoramic radiography. *Oral Radiology, 36*, 337–343.
45. Johari, M., Esmaeili, F., Andalib, A., et al. (2017). Detection of vertical root fractures in intact and endodontically treated premolar teeth by designing a probabilistic neural network: An ex vivo study. *Dentomaxillofacial Radiology, 46*, 20160107.

46. Seidberg, B. H., Alibrandi, B. V., Fine, H., & Logue, B. (1975). Clinical investigation of measuring working lengths of root canals with an electronic device and with digital-tactile sense. *Journal of the American Dental Association, 90*, 379–387.
47. Connert, T., Hülber, J. M., Godt, A., et al. (2014). Accuracy of endodontic working length determination using cone beam computed tomography. *International Endodontic Journal, 47*, 698–703.
48. Serna-Peña, G., Gomes-Azevedo, S., Flores-Treviño, J., et al. (2020). In vivo evaluation of 3 electronic apex locators: Root ZX Mini, Apex ID, and Propex Pixi. *Journal of Endodontics, 46*, 158–161.
49. Saghiri, M. A., Asgar, K., Boukani, K. K., et al. (2012). A new approach for locating the minor apical foramen using an artificial neural network. *International Endodontic Journal, 45*, 257–265.
50. Petersson, A., Axelsson, S., Davidson, T., et al. (2012). Radiological diagnosis of periapical bone tissue lesions in endodontics: A systematic review. *International Endodontic Journal, 45*, 783–801.
51. Tewary, S., Luzzo, J., & Hartwell, G. (2011). Endodontic radiography: Who is reading the digital radiograph? *Journal of Endodontics, 37*, 919–921.
52. Saghiri, M. A., Garcia-Godoy, F., Gutmann, J. L., et al. (2012). The reliability of artificial neural network in locating minor apical foramen: A cadaver study. *Journal of Endodontics, 38*, 1130–1134.
53. Hiraiwa, T., Ariji, Y., Fukuda, M., et al. (2019). A deep-learning artificial intelligence system for assessment of root morphology of the mandibular first molar on panoramic radiography. *Dentomaxillofacial Radiology, 48*, 20180218.
54. Christodoulou, A., Mikrogeorgis, G., Vouzara, T., et al. (2018). A new methodology for the measurement of the root canal curvature and its 3D modification after instrumentation. *Acta Odontologica Scandinavica, 76*, 488–492.
55. Gu, D., Liang, C., & Zhao, H. (2017). A case-based reasoning system based on weighted heterogeneous value distance metric for breast cancer diagnosis. *Artificial Intelligence in Medicine, 77*, 31–47.
56. Campo, L., Aliaga, I. J., De Paz, J. F., et al. (2016). Retreatment predictions in odontology by means of CBR systems. *Computational Intelligence and Neuroscience, 2016*, 7485250.
57. Aminoshariae, A., Kulild, J., & Nagendrababu, V. (2021). Artificial intelligence in endodontics: Current applications and future directions. *Journal of Endodontics, 47*(9), 1352–1357. https://doi.org/10.1016/j.joen.2021.06.003.

CHAPTER 7

Teknomo–Fernandez Kernelized Discriminant Analysis-Based Connectionist Deep Multilayer Perceptive Neural Learning for Human Activity Recognition

R. BAGAVATHI LAKSHMI[1] and A. SARANYA[2]

[1]*Assistant Professor, Department of Computer Applications, Mannar Thirumalai Naicker College, Tamil Nadu, India*

[2]*Guest Lecturer, Department of Computer Applications, Madurai Kamaraj University, Tamil Nadu, India*

ABSTRACT

Human activity recognition is one of the upcoming types of research in recent days for identification of the movement or action of a person depending on variety of sensor data. Although much of the work has been done on human activity recognition but accurate recognition is the main issue due to the complexity and uncertainty of real scenarios. A novel technique called Teknomo–Fernandez kernelized discriminant Feature based Connectionist deep multilayer perceptive neural learning (TFKDF-CDMPNL) has improved the accuracy in human activity detection to a great extent. The activity is monitored by fitting the wearable sensors in the human body and then storing the dataset pertaining to human activity. The dataset is multivariate and neural networks are used to train the model. Basically, the Multilayer Perceptron with input,

Data-Driven Analytics for Healthcare: Artificial Intelligence and Machine Learning for Medical Diagnostics. Meghna Sharma, Priyanka Vashisht, A. V. Senthil Kumar, Chitra Singh, and Abdelmalek Amine (Eds.)

hidden, and output layer is used. Multiple video sequences are taken as input-by-input layer and then transferred to first hidden layer where they are packaged into frames. Teknomo–Fernandez algorithm determines foreground and background frames after separating them. After that the Radial basis kernelized discriminant Feature extraction process is carried out for finding important and robust features so that the process of human activity recognition be done in optimal time. The last layer is used for classification and Czekanowski dice similarity coefficient is used to analyze features and final classification. The similarity value is studied by using binary step activation function with threshold value. The results shown by TFKDF-CDMPML have been remarkably accurate for human activity recognition activity. Accuracy, precision, recall, F-measure, and time complexity with respect to the number of video sequences are some of the performance measures used to check the performance and based on the results the proposed TFKDF-CDMPNL technique has shown improvement in the performance of human action recognition accuracy with lesser time consumption.

7.1 INTRODUCTION

Human Activity Recognition (HAR) is the process of automatically detecting a variety of physical activities performed by people in their day-to-day lives. HAR is a significant and challenging topic due to the tasks being repeated several times by humans. This is motivated by providing classification and robust validation, as well as test approaches for accurate recognition. However, accurate evaluation is difficult due to the time consumption.

A hybrid deep domain adaptation neural network (HydraNet) was developed by Aria et al. [1] for identifying human activities. However, the designed technique increased accuracy, but robust features were not extracted to minimize time complexity. A Gaussian Mixture Model, Kalman Filter, and Gated Recurrent Neural Network (GMM+KF+GRNN) were developed by Neziha et al. [2] for detecting human actions with higher accuracy. The designed method failed to evaluate our approach for minimizing the time of video classification.

A feed-forward learning model was developed by Nudrat Nida, Muhammad et al. [3] for activity recognition with higher accuracy.

However, complexity analysis was not performed. A deep residual neural network using convolutional layers was developed by Minhyuk & Seokho [4] to categorize activities with less time. However, the accuracy was not improved. A Generative Adversarial Nets (GAN)-based augmentation neural network was developed by Junhao et al. [5] for classifying certain activities. However, the developed network did not reduce time consumption.

A deep recurrent model was developed by Jianchao et al. [6] for identifying human activities. However, the designed model was not efficient in accurately recognizing human activities in less time. A convolutional neural network (CNN) was developed by Shaohua et al. [7] for real-time human activity classification by extracting high-efficiency features. However, the foreground and background frame extraction process was not carried out to reduce complexity. A Stacking Denoising Autoencoder and Light GBM (LGB) were developed by Xile et al. [8] for identifying humans by extracting more efficient features. The developed methods did not achieve higher recognition accuracy in minimum time. Transfer learning with fine-tuning techniques was introduced by Saeedeh et al. [9] for human activities based on frame sequences. Multi-Label Classification was performed by Manan et al. [10] to handle the complex problem of multi-resident activity recognition. However, the technique consumed more time to perform Multi-Label Classification.

7.2 OUR CONTRIBUTIONS

The main contribution of the proposed TFKDF-CDMPNL work is summarized as given below:

- To increase the human activity recognition accuracy, a novel TFKDF-CDMPNL technique is introduced based on the Connectionist deep multilayer perceptron neural learning.
- To minimize the time and space complexity, Teknomo–Fernandez foreground detection and Radial basis kernelized discriminant feature extraction processes are carried out. The Teknomo–Fernandez algorithm selects the foreground frame and removes the background frames. Then the robust features are extracted from the foreground frames.

- To increase the accuracy, Czekanowski's dice similarity is applied to analyze the features with their respective classes. Based on the similarity value, binary step activation is applied to recognize the human activity. This helps to reduce the false positive rate.
- Finally, an extensive simulation is conducted to estimate the performance of our TFKDF-CDMPNL technique and other related works. The results demonstrate that our TFKDF-CDMPNL technique is highly efficient compared to other methods.

7.3 ORGANIZATION

The rest of the chapter is arranged into different sections as follows: Section 7.2 discusses the related works. Section 7.3 provides the methodology of research in detail. Section 7.4 describes the experimental evaluation. Section 7.5 discusses the results with different performance metrics. Finally, Section 7.6 summarizes the conclusions for this research work.

7.4 RELATED WORKS

The hidden conditional random fields (HCRFs) were developed by Muhammad et al. [3] for human activity recognition. However, it failed to minimize the recognition time when employed in a real environment. A statistical weighted segmentation and rank correlation-based method was developed by Muhammad et al. [11] for feature selection to increase classification accuracy. However, the false positive rate was not minimized. A hierarchical multi-view aggregation system was developed by Xiheng et al. [12] based on multi-view feature spaces to increase the accuracy of activity recognition. However, it was not applicable for sensor-based human activity recognition.

An information theory was developed by Hendrio & Juan [13] for human activity recognition by extracting features with lower computational cost. A capsule network was designed by Cuong et al. [14] to identify human activity from wearable sensors using spatio-temporal data. However, complexity analysis was not performed. A global method was developed by Kévin et al. [15] based on probabilistic finite-state automata to increase recognition performance with lower computational complexity.

A hybrid deep learning network was developed by Tianqi et al. [16] for human activity recognition. However, accurate recognition was not achieved. Personalization models were developed by Anna et al. [17] to improve the accuracy of machine learning algorithms for activity recognition. A fully Distributed Collaborative Reasoning (DCR) model was developed by Amina et al. [18] to improve their own performance in activity recognition. A deep learning multi-channel architecture was developed by Sibor et al. [19] by integrating the convolutional neural network (CNN) and Bidirectional Long Short-Term Memory (BLSTM) for activity recognition.

7.5 PROPOSAL METHODOLOGY

The proposed TFKDF-CDMPNL technique is introduced in order to design an efficient human recognition system with higher accuracy and lesser time consumption. The proposed TFKDF-CDMPNL technique uses feature extraction and classification. Connectionist Deep Multilayer Perceptron is a type of machine learning algorithm inspired by the structure and function of the brain called artificial neural networks. The deep learning algorithm comprises different layers for learning the given input sequences. The proposed technique exactly recognizes the input with a minimal error rate when compared to existing works. The architecture diagram of the proposed TFKDF-CDMPNL technique is depicted in Figure 7.1.

Figure 7.1 portrays the architecture diagram of the proposed TFKDF-CDMPNL technique consisting of two major processes such as feature extraction and classification for improving human activity recognition with higher accuracy. The human activities are recorded in the videos. The numerous videos $V=v_1, v_2, v_3, \ldots. v_n$ are collected from the dataset '*D*.' In the data acquisition process, multiple video sequences are collected from the dataset.

Figure 7.2 portrays the schematic representation of connectionist deep multilayer perceptron learning which comprises neuron-like nodes positioned into different layers. In the connectionist method, the nodes are connected to construct the networks. The structure of the connections varies from design to design. The proposed deep learning concept uses a feed-forward network where the input data is processed in the forward

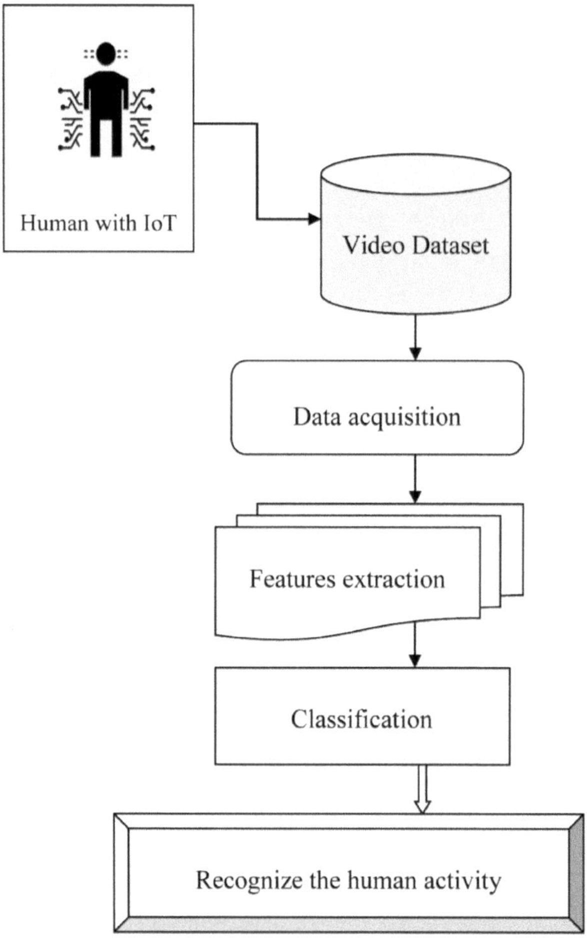

FIGURE 7.1 Architecture of the proposed TFKDF-CDMPNL technique.

direction. Here, the feed-forward deep structure learning framework connects the input from the previous layer to the consecutive layer. The architecture consists of three layers: input layer, hidden layers, and output layer. The input layer supplies the input to the hidden layer for calculations and manipulations. Then, the hidden layers process the given input and forward it to the output layer, which produces the classification results. Based on the classification results, human activities are correctly recognized. Therefore, the proposed architecture automatically learns the given input based on a layer-by-layer method.

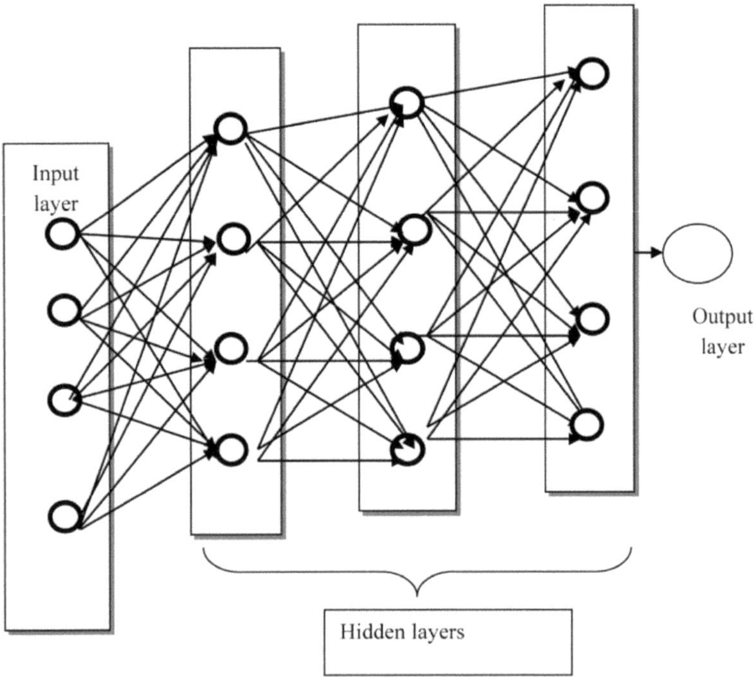

FIGURE 7.2 Schematic representation of connectionist deep multilayer perceptive neural learning.

Let us consider the number of video sequences $V=v_1,v_2,v_3,....v_n$ is given to the input layer. The activity of the neuron at the input layer as given below:

$$Q(t) = c + \sum_{i=1}^{n} V_i(t) * \delta_1 \quad (1)$$

From (), Q(t) denotes an activity of the neuron, 'V_i(t) ' indicates a input, i.e., video sequences $V=v_1,v_2,v_3,....v_n$, 'δ_1' indicates a weight to strengthen the connections between the layers, 'c' represents a bias and it stored the value is 1. The input is transferred into the first hidden layer where the frame detection is performed.

7.5.1 TEKNOMO–FERNANDEZ-BASED FOREGROUND DETECTION

The first process of proposed TFKDF-CDMPNL technique is to perform the frame detection using Teknomo–Fernandez algorithm for generating the background image and foreground images of a given video sequence. Initially, the input video sequences are partitioned into different frames $F=f_1,v_2,f_3,\ldots,f_n$. Then the foreground detection process is performed by subtracting the background image from the original image for accurate activity recognition. Let us consider the video frame as input, the pixel values, i.e., integer of frames converts into the bit level representation. Let us consider bit level representation of three frames b_1,b_2,b_3. Therefore, the background of the image is obtained as follows:

$$B = b_3\left(b_1 \oplus b_2\right) + b_1 b_2 \tag{2}$$

where; B denotes a background image. Then the Boolean mode function (F) is applied to differentiate the background and foreground.

$$F = \begin{cases} 1 \; ; & \sum_{i=1}^{n} b_i \geq \left(\frac{n}{2}+1\right) \quad where\ n = \geq 3 \\ 0 \; ; & \qquad Otherwise \end{cases} \tag{3}$$

Where n denotes a number of frames. From the above equation, the Boolean function returns '1' indicates that the background; otherwise, it indicates that the foreground. By applying the above equation, the foreground and background images are correctly identified. The foreground frame is chosen for further processing, i.e., feature extraction and classification. Whereas the background frames are removed. This process minimizes the time consumption of human activity recognition.

7.5.2 RADIAL BASIS KERNELIZED DISCRIMINANT ANALYSIS FEATURE EXTRACTION

The second process is to perform the feature extraction from the selected foreground video frames. The features play a very significant role in human activity recognition with minimum time consumption. Therefore, the proposed technique uses Radial basis kernelized discriminant function to find a projection for the features into a lower dimensional space. Here, the Radial basis kernel function is used to measure the similarity between the mean of the subset and the features. The similarity is measured as given below:

$$K = e(-\frac{1}{2d^2} \| f_i - m \|^2) \tag{4}$$

From (), K denotes a kernel function, f_i signifies a feature set, m indicates a mean, d denotes a deviation parameter. $|f_i\_m\|^2$ represents the squared Euclidean distance between the feature and the mean. The minimum distance between the features and the mean is selected as robust features from small sequence of poses. In this way, the robust features get extracted in effective manner for accurately recognizing the human activity. Then the extracted robust features are sent to the next hidden layer.

7.5.3 CZEKANOWSKI'S DICE SIMILARITY

Finally, the classification is performed based on the Czekanowski's dice similarity for identifying the different human activities. Let us consider the robust features $RF=rf_1, rf_2, ...rf_n$, and the number of classes $c_1, c_2, c_3, ... c_k$, . Then the similarity between the features and classes are measured as given below:

$$R = 1 - 2 * \left[\frac{rfi \cap c_j}{rfi \cup c_j} \right] \tag{5}$$

where; R represents a Czekanowski's dice similarity coefficient; rf_i denotes robust features in the dataset; c_j denotes a class. From Eqn. (5), the intersection symbol '∩' indicates a mutual dependence between robust features and the classes; and the union symbol 'U' signifies all features. The similarity coefficient (R) provides the integer value in the range from 0 to 1. The output of hidden layer is represented as follows:

$$W(t) = [\Sigma_{i=1}^{n} V_i(t) * \delta_1] + [\delta_2 * Wt - 1] \tag{6}$$

where; W(t) indicates an output of hidden layer at a time 't',; δ_1 represents a weight value between input and hidden layer; $V_i(t)$ represents the input; δ_2 indicates a weight of hidden layers; V_{t-1} denotes an output of the previous hidden layer. Then the output is fed into the output layer.

$$Y(t) = \sigma_b\{\delta_3 * W(t)\} \tag{7}$$

From Eqn. (7), '$Y(t)$ denote the output of the deep neural network at the time 't,' δ_3 denotes a weight between the hidden and output layer, $W(t)$ indicates an output of the hidden layer, σ_b denotes a binary step activation function. In the output layer, the classification results are obtained using binary step activation function. The activation function analyzes the similarity value and returns outcomes either '1' or '0.'

$$\sigma_b = \begin{cases} R > T; & retuns\, 1 \\ Otherwise; & retuns\, 0 \end{cases} \tag{8}$$

Where; R denotes a similarity; T indicates a threshold; σ_b denotes a binary step activation function. If the similarity value is higher than the threshold, then the sequence is classified into the particular class. In this way, the given input sequence is correctly classified into different classes. Based on the classification results, the human activities are correctly recognized with higher accuracy. The algorithm process of the proposed TFKDF-CDMPNL technique is described as follows:

\\ **Algorithm 1:**
Input: Video dataset 'D,' videos '$V=v_1, v_2, \ldots. v_n$'
Output: Increase Human activity recognition accuracy

Begin:

1. Collect the number of videos '$V=v_1, v_2, \ldots. v_n$' at input layer

// **hidden Layer 1**

2. For each 'v_i'
3. Divide into number of frames $F=f_1, v_2, f_3, \ldots, f_n$
4. For each frame 'f_i'
5. Measure background of the image 'B'
6. If $F=1$ then
7. Frame is said to be a foreground
8. Else
9. Frame is said to be a background
10. Else if
11. Select foreground frames
12. Remove background frames
13. End for
14. End for

// **hidden Layer 2**

15. For each feature

$$K = e(-\frac{1}{2d^2} \| f_i - m \|^2)$$

16. Measure similarity
17. Extract robust features
18. End for

// hidden Layer 3
Initialize the number of classes $c_1, c_2, c_3, \ldots. c_k$,
For each class c_i
For each robust feature rf_1
Measure similarity 'R' and sent to the output layer

// Output Layer
If (R>T) then
σ_b returns '1'
Classify sequence into particular class
Else
σ_b returns '0'
End if
End

The step-by-step process of the proposed TFKDF-CDMPNL technique is described for increasing the human activity recognition accuracy with lesser time consumption. The deep learning method comprises different layers to learn the given input video sequences. In the first hidden layer, the video sequences are partitioned into different frames and the foreground video frame is detected by applying the Teknomo–Fernandez algorithm. The background frames are removed to minimize the complexity of activity recognition. After finding the foreground frame, the feature extraction process is performed by applying the Radial basis kernelized discriminant analysis. The radial basis kernel function measures the correlation between the feature and the mean value. Followed by the robust features are correctly identified at the second hidden layer. Then the extracted feature is sent to the third hidden layer for classifying the video sequences. The Czekanowski's dice index is applied to measure the similarity between the robust features and classes. Finally, the similarity value is transferred to the output layer. The binary step activation function is used to analyze the similarity value and return the classification results at the output layer. This helps to accurately recognize human activities and minimize the false positive rate.

7.6 EXPERIMENTAL SETUP

The proposed TFKDF-CDMPNL and two existing methods, namely HydraNet by Tran & Sorokin [20] and GMM+KF+GRNN, are implemented in the JAVA platform using the UIUC action dataset by Tran &

Sorokin. The main aim of the dataset is to recognize human activities such as walking, running, jumping, waving, jumping jacks, clapping, jumping from sit up, raising one hand, stretching out, turning, sitting to standing, crawling, pushing up, and standing sitting. From the dataset, 200 video sequences are taken to conduct the experiments for 10 runs. For each run, various counts of inputs are taken in the form of 20, 40, 60, 80, …, 100. Different evaluation metrics are used to analyze the performance of the TFKDF-CDMPNL technique and existing methods. The parameters include human activity recognition accuracy, false positive rate, human activity recognition time, and space complexity.

7.6.1 HUMAN ACTIVITY RECOGNITION ACCURACY

The human activity recognition accuracy is measured as the ratio of the number of sequences correctly recognized to the total number of sequences taken for conducting the experiments. The formula for calculating the accuracy is expressed as given below:

$$HARA = \left(\frac{Number\ of\ correctly\ recognized\ sequences}{Total\ number\ of\ sequences}\right) * 100 \tag{9}$$

where; *HARA* indicates a human activity recognition accuracy which is measured in terms of percentage (%).

7.6.2 FALSE POSITIVE RATE

The human activity recognition accuracy is measured as the ratio of the number of sequences wrongly recognized to the total number of sequences. The false positive rate is mathematically calculated as follows:

$$FPR = \left(\frac{NSWR}{n}\right) * 100 \tag{10}$$

where; *FPR* indicates a false positive rate; *NSWR* denotes a number of sequences wrongly recognized; '*n*' indicates a number of sequences. The false positive rate is measured in terms of percentage (%).

7.6.3 HUMAN ACTIVITY RECOGNITION TIME

The human activity recognition time is measured as an amount of time taken by the algorithm to recognize the human activities based on the classification. The mathematical formula for calculating the time is expressed as follows:

$$HART = Number\ of\ sequences * Time\left(to\, recognize\, the\, one\, sequences\right) \quad (11)$$

where; *HART* represent human activity recognition time is calculated in terms of milliseconds (ms).

7.6.4 SPACE COMPLEXITY

The space complexity is measured as an amount of memory space consumed by the algorithm to store the different sequences. The mathematical formula for calculating the time is expressed as follows:

$$SC = n * M\left(recognized\ one\ sequences\right) \quad (12)$$

where; *SC* represent space complexity; '*n*' denotes a number of sequences; M indicates a memory space. The space complexity is calculated in terms of kilobytes (KB).

7.7 RESULTS AND DISCUSSION

The experimental results of TFKDF-CDMPNL and two existing methods, namely HydraNet and GMM+KF+GRNN, are discussed based on various performance metrics such as human activity recognition accuracy, false positive rate, human activity recognition time, and space complexity. The performance results are discussed and compared with the help of tables and graphical representations.

Table 7.1 shows the experimental results of Human activity recognition accuracy using three different methods namely TFKDF-CDMPNL and two existing methods namely Hydra Net, GMM+KF+GRNN. As shown in Table 7.1, 10 different results are obtained for each method based on the input counts 20, 40, 60, 80, ... 200. The observed results indicate that the accuracy of TFKDF-CDMPNL technique is higher than the other two conventional methods. This is proved through the statistical results. Let us consider 20 video sequences taken from the dataset for conducting the experiments. By applying the TFKDF-CDMPNL technique, 16 sequences are correctly recognized hence the accuracy is 80%. Whereas 15 and 14 sequences are correctly detected by using Hydra Net, GMM+KF+GRNN and their accuracy percentages are 75% and 70%, respectively. Similarly, 10 results are observed for each method. Finally, the average of 10 results indicates that the human recognition accuracy is considerably increased by 5% and 9% when compared to existing Hydra Net, GMM+KF+GRNN, respectively.

TABLE 7.1 Human Activity Recognition Accuracy

Number of Sequences	Human Activity Recognition Accuracy (%)		
	TFKDF-CDMPNL	Hydra Net	GMM+KF+GRNN
20	80	75	70
40	80	80	75
60	83	80	77
80	85	81	79
100	87	83	80
120	90	86	83
140	92	88	86
160	93	89	87
180	96	89	87
200	98	90	88

Figure 7.3 shows the performance results of Human activity recognition accuracy of different methods. In the chart, the number of input video sequences is shown on the horizontal axis and the accuracy results are displayed on the vertical axis. The accuracy of different methods is represented by three different colors of columns: blue, green, and red. The graphical plot indicates that the proposed TFKDF-CDMPNL technique provides superior performance in terms of achieving higher accuracy. This is attributed to the application of the Connectionist deep multilayer perceptron neural learning in TFKDF-CDMPNL technique. The deep perceptron learning analyzes the robust features extracted from the video frames. Then, Czekanowski's dice function is applied to measure the similarity between the features and the classes. Based on the similarity measure, the video sequences are correctly categorized into different classes.

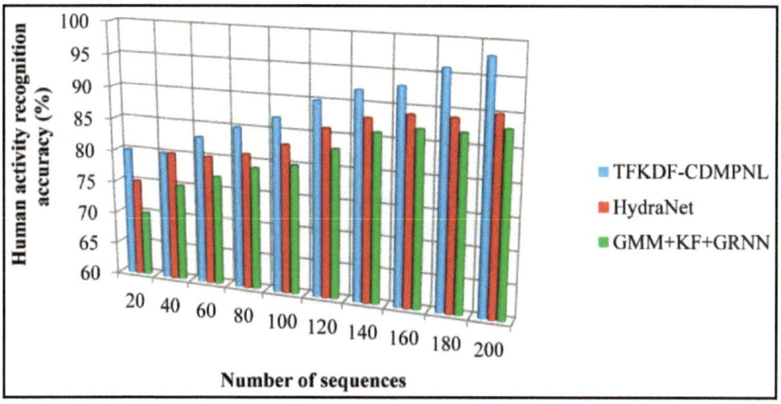

FIGURE 7.3 Graphical representation of human activity recognition accuracy.

Experimental results of the false positive rate of human activity recognition of three different techniques, namely TFKDF-CDMPNL, and two existing methods, namely HydraNet and GMM+KF+GRNN, are described in Table 7.2. The false positive rate is measured based on the number of video sequences taken in the ranges from 20 to 200. The observed results indicate that the incorrect classification is minimized when compared to existing methods. In the first iteration, 20 video sequences are considered, and the false positive rate is 20%. By applying HydraNet and GMM+KF+GRNN, false positive rates of 25% and 30% are observed. Subsequently, nine runs are carried out for each method, and the average results indicate that the false positive rate of the proposed TFKDF-CDMPNL technique is considerably minimized by 33% and 43%, respectively.

TABLE 7.2 False Positive Rate

Number of Sequences	False Positive Rate (%)		
	TFKDF-CDMPNL	Hydra Net	GMM+KF+GRNN
20	20	25	30
40	20	23	25
60	17	20	23
80	15	19	21
100	13	17	20
120	10	14	17
140	8	12	14.
160	7	11	13
180	4	11	13
200	2	10	12

Figure 7.4 demonstrates the experimental results of false positive rate according to the number of video sequences. As shown in the graph, the number of video sequences is taken as input for calculating the false positive rate. The results show that the proposed TFKDF-CDMPNL technique achieves a lower false positive rate than the existing methods. This is due to the application of Czekanowski's Dice index to the TFKDF-CDMPNL technique to evaluate the similarity between the robust features and classes. Finally, the similarity value is sent to the output layer where the binary step activation function is applied to analyze the similarity value with the threshold. The classification results are then obtained at the output layer, reducing incorrect recognition.

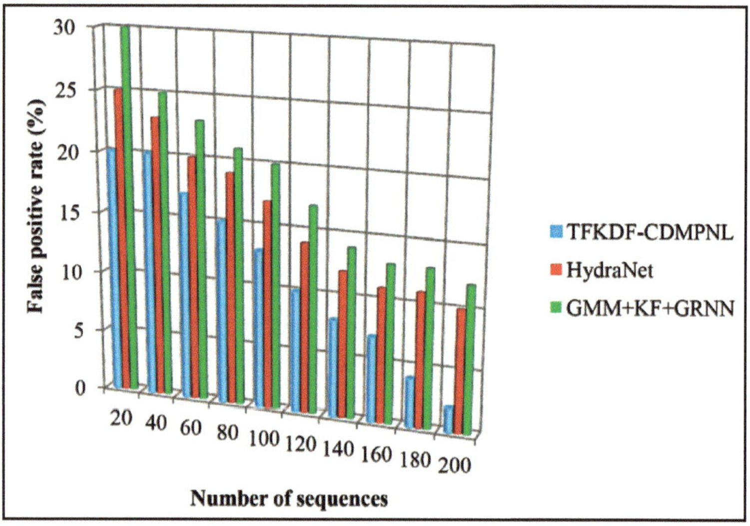

FIGURE 7.4 Graphical representation of false positive rate.

Table 7.3 describes the experimental results of human activity recognition time versus the number of video sequences. Thus, the time consumption of the TFKDF-CDMPNL is considerably reduced compared to conventional methods. Additionally, from the sample calculation provided in Table 7.3, when 'video sequences' are considered, the time consumption for classifying the given sequence using the TFKDF-CDMPNL technique was found to be "14*ms*" and the space complexity of HydraNet, GMM+KF+GRNN was found to be "16*ms* " and "18*ms*," respectively. The overall observed results show that human activity recognition time is considerably reduced by 11% and 20% using the TFKDF-CDMPNL technique when compared to conventional methods.

TABLE 7.3 Human Activity Recognition Time

Number of Sequences	Human Activity Recognition Time (ms)		
	TFKDF-CDMPNL	HydraNet	GMM+KF+GRNN
20	14	16	18
40	15	17	20
60	16	18	21
80	17	19	22
100	18	20	22
120	19	22	24
140	20	23	25
160	21	24	26
180	23	25	27
200	26	28	30

The performance results of human activity recognition time along with the number of video sequences are illustrated in Figure 7.5. As shown in the graphic representation, the recognition time gradually increases for all the methods as the number of video sequences increases, since the count of inputs increases for each run. Additionally, a linear increasing trend can be observed. The observed results show that the recognition time is reduced by applying the TFKDF-CDMPNL technique. Initially, the input video sequences are converted into a number of frames, and the foreground frames are identified, and the other frames are removed using

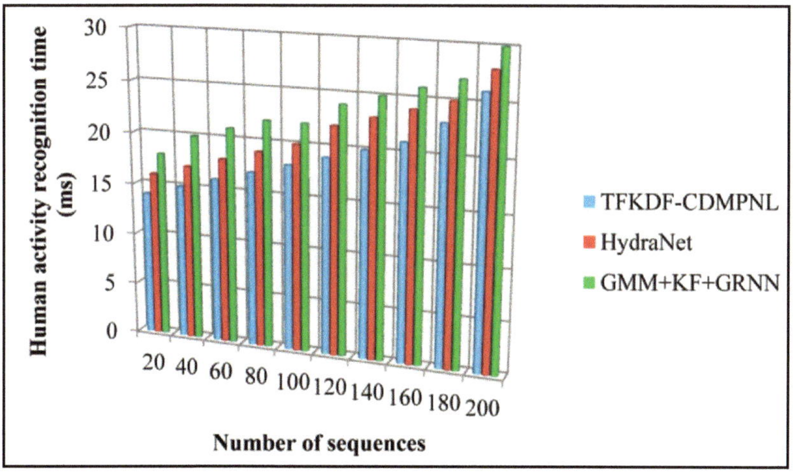

FIGURE 7.5 Graphical representation of human activity recognition time.

the Teknomo-Fernandez algorithm. This helps to reduce the complexity of activity recognition. Furthermore, the feature extraction process is performed by applying Radial Basis Kernelized Discriminant Analysis to extract robust features. With the extracted features, the classification is performed, resulting in a reduction of the recognition time.

Table 7.4 and Figure 7.6 demonstrate the performance results of the space complexity of three different methods, namely the TFKDF-CDMPNL technique, HydraNet, and GMM+KF+GRNN. The observed results indicate that the space complexity of the TFKDF-CDMPNL technique is considerably reduced compared to the other two methods. Let us consider 20 video sequences; the memory consumption for storing the given input sequence is using the TFKDF-CDMPNL technique. Similarly, the memory for storing the video sequences using HydraNet, GMM+KF+GRNN was found to be "1600 *KB*" and "1640 *KB* ," respectively. The overall observed results specify that the average space complexity is minimized by 5% and 11% using the TFKDF-CDMPNL technique when compared to conventional methods. It is inferred that the overall space complexity is considerably minimized using the TFKDF-CDMPNL technique by applying foreground frame detection and feature extraction. First, the video frames are divided into frames. Only the foreground frames are used to identify human activity; hence the background frames are removed. This results in lesser memory consumption. Besides, only the robust features are selected for classification, which also reduces the memory space.

TABLE 7.4 Space Complexity

Number of Sequences	Space Complexity (KB)		
	TFKDF-CDMPNL	HydraNet	GMM+KF+GRNN
20	1520	1600	1640
40	1760	1840	1920
60	1800	1920	2100
80	2000	2080	2240
100	2100	2200	2400
120	2280	2400	2520
140	2310	2450	2660
160	2400	2560	2720
180	2484	2610	2844
200	2520	2700	2920

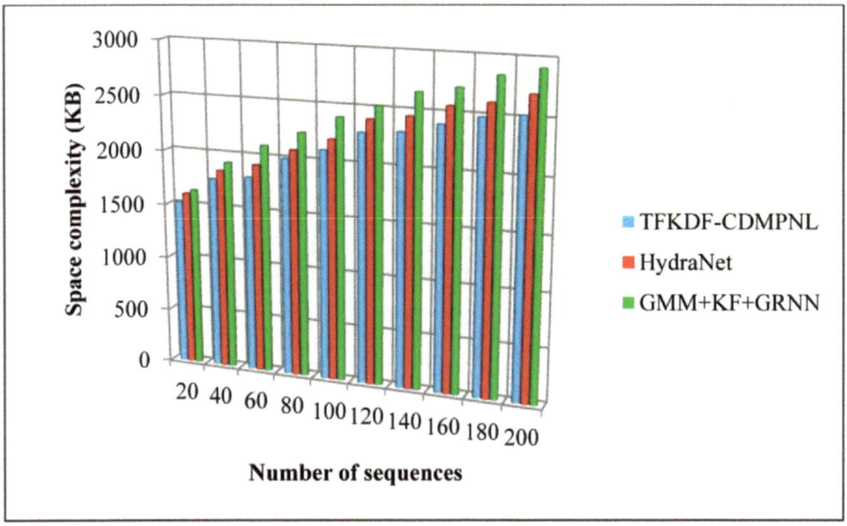

FIGURE 7.6 Graphical representation of space complexity.

7.8 CONCLUSION

In this chapter, a novel TFKDF-CDMPNL technique is introduced for human activity recognition with higher accuracy and less time consumption. The Connectionist deep multilayer perceptron neural learning analyzes the given input video frames using many layers. The Teknomo–Fernandez algorithm is applied to the hidden layer for detecting the foreground and background frames. Following that, Radial basis kernelized discriminant robust feature extraction process is carried out in the TFKDF-CDMPNL technique to minimize time and space consumption. Finally, the classification is performed at the third hidden layer using Czekanowski's dice similarity. At the output layer, a binary step activation function is applied to analyze the similarity value with the threshold value. As a result, the classification outcomes are observed at the output layer with higher accuracy. An experimental evaluation is conducted for the TFKDF-CDMPNL technique and existing methods with different performance metrics. The discussed results indicate that the proposed TFKDF-CDMPNL technique outperforms well in terms of achieving higher human activity recognition accuracy and minimum false positives, time, and space complexity than the other conventional methods.

KEYWORDS

- **binary step activation function**
- **connectionist deep multilayer perceptive neural learning**
- **Czekanowski's dice similarity**
- **human activity recognition**
- **radial basis kernelized discriminant feature extraction**
- **Teknomo-Fernandez algorithm**

REFERENCES

1. Aria, G. P., Bernardo, N. Y., & Seok-Lyong, L. (2020). Hybrid domain adaptation with deep network architecture for end-to-end cross-domain human activity recognition. *Computers & Industrial Engineering*, 1–9. Elsevier.
2. Neziha, J., Noureddine, B., & Med. S. B. (2020). A new hybrid deep learning model for human action recognition. *Journal of King Saud University – Computer and Information Sciences*, *32*(4), 447–453. Elsevier.
3. Muhammad, H., Madallah, A., Amjad, A., Saad, A., & Furkh, Z. (2019). Human activity recognition using Gaussian mixture hidden conditional random fields. *Computational Intelligence and Neuroscience*, 1–14. Hindawi.
4. Minhyuk, J., & Seokho, C. (2020). Human activity classification based on sound recognition and residual convolutional neural network. *Automation in Construction*, *114*, 1–10. Elsevier.
5. Junhao, S., Decheng, Z., & Zhan, Z. (2020). A GAN-based data augmentation method for human activity recognition via the caching ability. *Internet Technology Letters*, 1–8. Wiley.
6. Jianchao, L., Xi, Z., Michael, S., Jiong, J., & Shui, Y. (2020). Efficient human activity recognition using a single wearable sensor. *IEEE Internet of Things Journal*, *7*(11), 11137–11146.
7. Shaohua, W., Lianyong, Q., Xiaolong, X., Chao, T., & Gu, Z. (2020). Deep learning models for real-time human activity recognition with smartphones. *Mobile Networks and Applications*, *25*(3), 743–755. https://doi.org/10.1007/s11036-020-01517-7.
8. Xile, G., Haiyong, L., Fang, Z., Langlang, Y., & Yuexia, Z. (2019). A human activity recognition algorithm based on stacking denoising autoencoder and LightGBM. *Sensors*, *19*(1), 1–20. https://doi.org/10.3390/s19010151.
9. Saeedeh, Z., & Vahid, A. (2020). Human activity recognition by using MHIs of frame sequences. *Turkish Journal of Electrical Engineering & Computer Sciences*, 23, 1716–1730.

10. Manan, J., Abhishek, S., Thinagaran, P., & Jieh-Ren, C. (2020). Multi-label classification based ensemble learning for human activity recognition in smart home. *Internet of Things*, 12, 1–13. Elsevier.
11. Muhammad, S., Muhammad, A., Farooq, Z., Jamal, H., & Tallha, A. (2020). Human action recognition: A framework of statistical weighted segmentation and rank correlation-based selection. *Pattern Analysis and Applications*, 23, 281–294. Springer.
12. Xiheng, Z., Yongkang, W., Mohan, S. K., & Weidong, G. (2019). Hierarchical multi-view aggregation network for sensor-based human activity recognition. *PLoS ONE, 14*(9), e0222639. https://doi.org/10.1371/journal.pone.0222639.
13. Hendrio, B., Juan, G., Wesllen, S., & Eduardo, S. (2018). A smartphone lightweight method for human activity recognition based on information theory. *Sensors, 20,* 1–28.
14. Cuong, P., Son, N. T., Huy, T. Q., Son, T., Hai, V., Thanh-Hai, T., & Thi-Lan Le. (2020). Sens CapsNet: Deep neural network for non-obtrusive sensing based human activity recognition. *IEEE Access, 8*, 86934–86946.
15. Kévin, V., Maria, P., Gregory, F., & Jean-Jacques, L. (2020). Human activity discovery and recognition using probabilistic finite-state automata. *IEEE Transactions on Automation Science and Engineering, 17*(4), 2085–2096.
16. Tianqi, L., & Xiaojuan, W. (2020). A hybrid network based on dense connection and weighted feature aggregation for human activity recognition. *IEEE Access, 8,* 68320–68332. https://doi.org/10.1109/ACCESS.2020.2986262.
17. Anna, F., Daniela, M., Marco, M., & Paolo, N. (2020). On the personalization of classification models for human activity recognition. *IEEE Access, 8*, 32066–32079.
18. Amina, J., Amel, B., & Khedija, A. (2020). DCR: A new distributed model for human activity recognition in smart homes. *Expert Systems with Applications, 140*, 1–51. Elsevier.
19. Sibor, K., Augustine, O., Solomon, H., Richard, I., Kayode, O., & Mobolaji, O. (2020). Deep learning approach for human activities recognition from multimodal sensing devices. *IEEE Access, 8,* 179028–179038. https://doi.org/10.1109/ACCESS.2020.3028423.
20. Tran, D., & Sorokin, A. (2008). Human activity recognition with metric learning. In *Proceedings of the 10th European Conference on Computer Vision (ECCV '08)* (pp. 548–561). Springer. https://doi.org/10.1007/978-3-540-88682-2_41.
21. Nudrat, N., Muhammad, H., Aun, I., & Sergio, A. V. (2019). Instructor activity recognition through deep spatiotemporal features and feedforward extreme learning machine. *Mathematical Problems in Engineering*, 1–13. Hindawi.

CHAPTER 8

Transforming Healthcare with AI: An Adequate Method for Diabetes Prediction Using Machine Learning Techniques

PRIYANKA SHARMA and MANI BUTWALL

Assistant Professor, Department of CSE, SKIT, Jaipur, Rajasthan, India

ABSTRACT

Artificial intelligence (AI) techniques, which are already widely employed in contemporary industry and daily life, are being used more and more in healthcare. Healthcare service providers may benefit from artificial intelligence in several regulatory processes and patient thought processes. Although the majority of AI and medical service innovations have a profound effect on the healthcare industry, the strategies they support can change significantly. Some review papers on AI in healthcare also suggest that AI may be able to diagnose diseases as well as or better than humans in some approaches. This chapter focuses on the healthcare impact of AI, the roles of AI in medical diagnosis, drug discovery, improving patient experience and healthcare workforce, AI's scaling in healthcare, and types of AI pertinent to healthcare. This chapter also considers efforts to plan and carry out a descriptive machine learning algorithm to create association standards to anticipate diabetes behavior in agreement with specific lifestyle characteristics, incorporating physical exercise and mental states, especially in older diabetics. The research emphasizes the Random Forest Classifier using the medical dataset from PIDD about the patients with

Data-Driven Analytics for Healthcare: Artificial Intelligence and Machine Learning for Medical Diagnostics.
Meghna Sharma, Priyanka Vashisht, A. V. Senthil Kumar, Chitra Singh, and Abdelmalek Amine (Eds.)

diabetic conditions. The correctness of the results with their statistical indicators is demonstrated through classification reports and confusion matrices.

8.1 INTRODUCTION

The healthcare industry is one of the biggest and most important in the world. Due to the recent COVID-19 crisis, this sector is currently the most crucial one, and it will continue to be at the forefront for a very long time. Healthcare could become better and more individualized while costing less due to advances in AI learning and suggestions as well as in diagnostics, sensors, and data analysis. The time has come for personalized health monitoring. The analytics, data, and recommendations help with the early identification and comprehension of health issues relating to chronic diseases and overall health/wellness. Diabetes, kidney disease, Parkinson's and Huntington's disorders, cardiovascular disease, cancer/oncology, and a wide range of other healthcare applications are a few examples.

Healthcare informatics is an interdisciplinary field that combines computer science, cognitive science, informatics concepts, information technology, and data science to address problems and support public health, medicine, healthcare, or regular health. In healthcare and medical domains, designing a trustworthy artificial intelligence (AI) solution is equally important if humans are to trust or regard these models as trustworthy [1]. In the healthcare sector, a paradigm shift toward healthcare 5.0 is projected. It utilizes patient-centered digital wellbeing and pushes the operational limits of healthcare 4.0. Healthcare 5.0 emphasizes ambient control, patient health tracking, welfare, and privacy compliance with the aid of technologies including AI, big data, IoT, etc. Figure 8.1 shows the areas of impact of AI in healthcare.

Artificial intelligence (AI) refers to the application of ML algorithms and various cognitive approaches in the healthcare industry. The simplest explanation of artificial intelligence is the capacity of computers or machines to replicate human learning, cognition, decision-making, and action (AI). In healthcare, AI relates to making use of machines for analyzing and performing actions on health data, with the objective of forecasting a particular outcome.

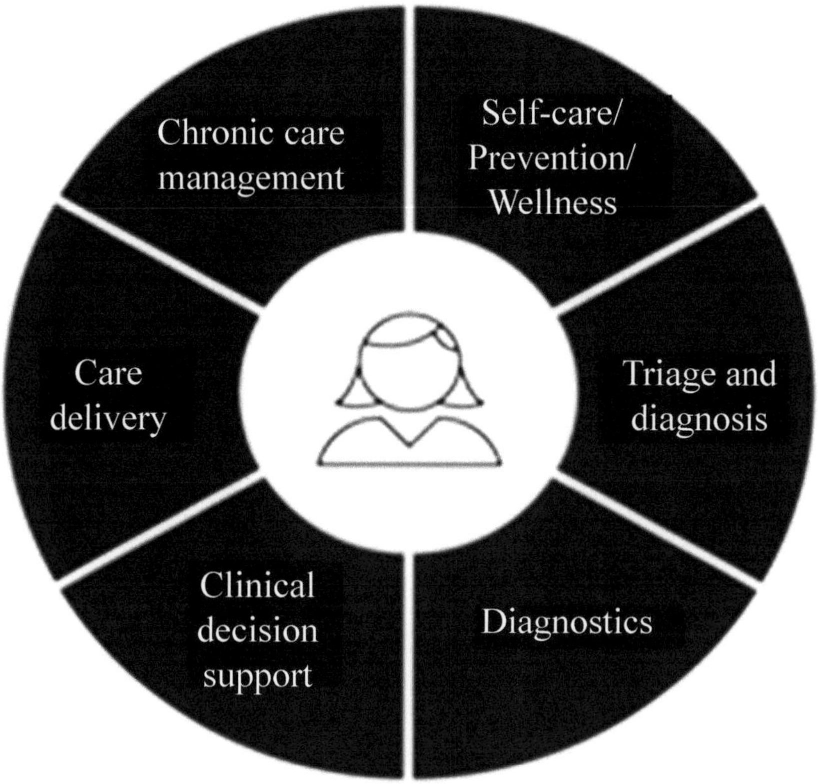

FIGURE 8.1 Areas of impacts of AI in healthcare.

Machine learning and other cognitive sciences are used for medical diagnostics, which is a significant use of AI in the healthcare industry. By leveraging patient data and related information, AI can assist physicians and other healthcare professionals in making diagnoses and treatment recommendations that are more accurate. By analyzing vast volumes of data to generate better preventive care ideas for patients, AI can also aid in making healthcare more predictive and proactive.

One of AI's greatest potential benefits is maintaining people's health so that they do not need to go to doctors regularly. AI, Internet of Medical Things, and consumer health applications help people adopt healthier behaviors and preventatively maintain a healthy lifestyle. Already, diseases like cancer are being more accurately and quickly diagnosed using AI [2].

AI has made mammogram reviews and interpretations 30 times faster and 99% correct, which eliminates the need for unnecessary biopsies. Utilizing cognitive technologies, healthcare organizations are leveraging IBM Watson for Health to access vast amounts of patient data and enable diagnosis. Figure 8.2 shows the worldwide market scenario for Artificial Intelligence.

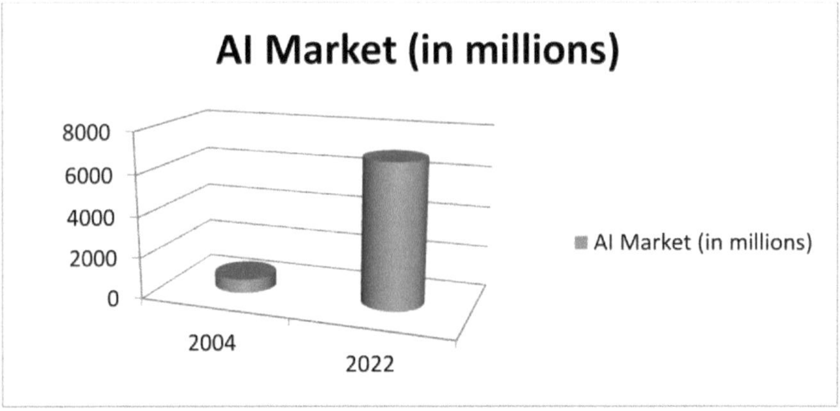

FIGURE 8.2 AI market worldwide, 2004–2022.

Google's DeepMind Health collaborates with physicians, patients, and researchers to address urgent healthcare concerns. By developing neural networks that closely mimic the human brain and incorporate effective algorithms, the technique integrates systems neuroscience and machine learning. Predictive analytics can help improve clinical decision-making and prioritize administrative responsibilities [3].

8.1.1 HEALTHCARE IMPACTS OF ARTIFICIAL INTELLIGENCE

The healthcare industry requires several important reforms. AI has the potential to drive advancements across the care continuum [4]. Patients have higher expectations of their healthcare providers, payment models are changing, and the amount of available data is growing rapidly. AI offers many advantages over clinical decision-making techniques and traditional analytics (Figure 8.3).

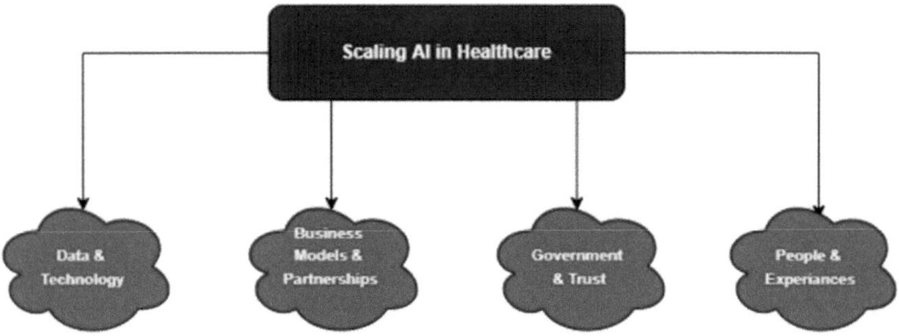

FIGURE 8.3 Scaling AI.

8.1.1.1 BROADCAST BETWEEN MACHINE AND MIND THROUGH BRAIN-COMPUTER INTERFACES

Although the idea of computer communication is by no means new, cutting-edge research is being done to bypass keyboards, mice, and monitors and connect technology and the human mind directly. For some patients, this research has significant ramifications. Due to neurological conditions and nervous system impairments, some people may lose the ability to move, speak, and participate effectively in social interactions with others and their environment. For many who believed they were lost forever, AI-powered brain-computer interfaces could restore those crucial experiences.

8.1.1.2 CREATING THE UP-AND-COMING RADIOLOGY EQUIPMENT

CT scanners, X-ray equipment, MRI machines create radiological images that all provide unobtrusive visibility in the human body. Various diagnostic methods continue to use real tissue samples from biopsies, which have risks like the potential for infection. According to scientists, the upcoming generation of radiological devices will be able to be more accurate and complete enough to occasionally replace the demand for tissue samples, thanks to artificial intelligence.

8.1.1.3 IMPROVING CARE ACCESS IN UNSERVED OR DEVELOPING REGIONS

Access to life-saving care can be severely constrained in undeveloped nations around the world due to a lack of qualified medical experts, such as radiologists and ultrasound technologists. The session mentioned that the 12 hospitals that compose Boston's renowned Longwood Avenue employ more radiologists than the whole of West Africa. AI may be able to mitigate the consequences of this severe scarcity of qualified clinical perpetrators by replacing some diagnostic duties traditionally performed by humans.

8.1.1.4 LOWERING THE BURDEN OF USE OF ELECTRONIC HEALTH RECORDS

The digitalization of the healthcare industry has been largely facilitated by EHRs, but it has also raised a variety of problems, such as customer burnout, unnecessary paperwork, and intellectual strain. EHR developers are using AI nowadays to build more user-friendly user interfaces and simplify some of the daily jobs that take up a lot of a user's time.

8.1.1.5 RESTRICTING ANTIBIOTIC RESISTANCE RISKS

Abuse of necessary drugs promotes the growth of superbugs that are resistant to treatments, posing a growing threat to societies worldwide. Multidrug resistant bacteria can wreak havoc in hospitals and cause hundreds of fatalities each year. Information from EHR can be used to pinpoint patients who are at risk for infection. By utilizing ML and AI tools, these insights may be made more precise, and notifications for healthcare providers can be sent out more quickly and accurately.

8.2 ADVANCES IN MEDICAL DIAGNOSIS OWING TO AI

8.2.1 VIZ.AI

To help care teams respond more rapidly in the healthcare sector, where delays can lead to the difference between death and life, Viz.ai offers AI-enabled healthcare remedies. Life-saving treatment decisions can be made by specialists thanks to the company's AI technology, which can quickly identify issues and warn care teams [5].

8.2.2 *FREENOME*

Freenome employs AI in blood tests, diagnostic procedures, and screenings to find cancer. The mission of Freenome is to find cancer in its initial stages and then provide innovative treatments.

8.2.3 *ENLITIC*

Enlitic develops deep learning medical solutions that expedite radiological diagnosis. Doctors may be able to better comprehend a patient's present needs with the use of the deep learning framework by analyzing ad-hoc medical data such as blood tests, radiological images, genomes, EKGs, and health records of patients.

8.2.4 *PATHAI*

PathAI creates ML for making more accurate diagnoses. The organization's current objectives include creating plans for individualized medical care and lowering the percentage of cancer detection errors. PathAI worked with organizations like the Bill & Melinda Gates Foundation and pharmaceutical corporations like Bristol-Myers Squibb to expand the use of their AI technology in the healthcare industry.

8.2.5 *BUOY HEALTH*

An AI-based tool that makes use of algorithms to detect and deal with ailments is known as Buoy Health. A chatbot will first inquire about a patient's symptoms and health concerns before rendering a diagnosis and directing them to the best care.

8.2.6 *ITERATIVE SCOPES*

By integrating AI with gastroenterology, Iterative Scopes enhances disease treatment and diagnosis. With the aid of AI, the company's AI Recruitment service automates the process of choosing individuals who are competent to participate in clinical trials for inflammatory bowel disease. The first clinical study of Iterative Scopes' AI-powered SKOUT device, which helps doctors discover potentially cancerous polyps, was also submitted for FDA evaluation.

8.3 EFFICIENCY OF AI IN DRUG DISCOVERY

Rising development costs and labor-intensive research are impeding the drug development business. Only 10% of drugs that undergo clinical trials are successfully commercialized, at an average cost of $1.3 billion [6]. Biopharmaceutical companies have quickly realized the effectiveness, precision, and comprehension that AI can provide thanks to technological advancements.

8.3.1 XTALPI

This platform combines cloud, AI, & quantum physics and forecasts the chemical and pharmacological properties of therapeutic candidates. The business also asserts that their crystal structure prediction technology anticipates complicated chemical systems in days as opposed to weeks or months. Investors in XtalPi have included Sequoia Capital, Google, and Tencent.

8.3.2 DEEP GENOMICS

Deep Genomics' AI platform makes it easier to find potential drug candidates to treat neurodegenerative and neuromuscular diseases. When the right candidates are found early in the development process, there is a statistically increased chance that a drug will pass clinical trials and that the time and cost to market will be reduced.

8.3.3 BENEVOLENT AI

Benevolent AI partners with major pharmaceutical firms to license goods in addition to collaborating with nonprofit organizations to offer transportable medication for rare diseases. Benevolent AI's main objective is to deliver the appropriate medicine to the appropriate patients at the appropriate time by utilizing AI to improve screening methods and deliver previously unrecognized insights through deep learning.

8.3.4 BIOXCEL

In the areas of immuno-oncology and neuroscience, AI is used by BioXcel Therapeutics to discover and develop new drugs. Companies use AI to identify new patients or develop creative uses for currently available medications.

8.3.5 BERG

To speed up the research and creation of revolutionary drugs, ailments are mapped at the clinical stage of the AI-based biotech platform BERG. BERG creates product candidates to treat uncommon diseases by fusing its "Interrogative Biology" technique with conventional R&D.

8.4 IMPROVEMENTS AI IS MAKING TO THE PATIENT EXPERIENCE

Time is money in the healthcare industry. Hospitals, clinics, and doctors can treat more patients each day by effectively delivering a smooth patient experience. In 2020, more than 33 million patients were admitted to U.S. hospitals, each with unique medical needs, insurance coverage, and circumstances that affected the quality of care [7]. According to studies, hospitals with satisfied patients make more money, while those with dissatisfied patients may suffer financial losses. The patient experience is being streamlined by new advancements in AI healthcare technologies, which are enabling medical staff to handle billions of data points more quickly and effectively.

8.4.1 OLIVE

Olive's AI platform automates routine medical tasks so that administrators can focus on more important ones. To free up staff members to concentrate on patient care, everything from eligibility verification through unresolved claims and data migrations is automated by the program.

8.4.2 QVENTUS INC

An AI-enabled software framework called Qventus addresses operational issues, such as those involving patient safety and emergency rooms. The company's software can map the quickest ambulance routes, manage hospital waiting times, and prioritize patient illness and injuries.

8.4.3 BABYLON

Babylon is on a mission to reengineer healthcare by changing the emphasis from treating the ill to preventing illness, which will result in improved health and lower medical costs.

8.4.4 TWIN HEALTH

Through a combination of AI, IoT technology, medical science, data science, and healthcare, this holistic approach aims to address and maybe repair chronic illnesses like Type 2 Diabetes. A digital representation of human metabolic function based on thousands of health data points, everyday activities, and individual preferences was developed by the business and named the Whole-Body Digital Twin.

8.4.5 SPRING HEALTH

Employers can use Spring Health's mental health benefit solution to provide their workforce with the resources to maintain good mental health. The clinically approved system collects each person's whole information and compares it to various thousands of data points. The software then matches users with the appropriate professional for face-to-face care or telemedicine appointments using ML.

8.4.6 KAIA HEALTH

To offer individuals care within the constraints of their schedules, Kaia Health runs a digital therapeutics platform with live physical therapists.

To treat COPD and chronic back pain, the platform offers individualized programs with case studies, workout plans, stress-relieving exercises, and learning resources.

8.5 AI'S IMPACT ON HEALTHCARE WORKFORCE

The MGI has investigated how AI and automation may change the nature of labor in the future. It is concluded that while automation will touch most employment across industries, the degree of impact will vary greatly [8]. Healthcare has one of the lowest overall automation potentials, with only 35% of time spent being automatable, depending on the vocation. The possibility of acceptance differs from the potential for automation. The analysis assumes a midway scenario that predicts that 15% of current healthcare labor hours would be automated. For a variety of healthcare vocations in a few European nations, the proportion of current work hours that automation could free up by 2030 [9] is shown in Exhibit 2. This does not consider the possibility of more disruption brought on by other elements, like personalization, which may completely transform healthcare by concentrating on a "segment of one."

8.6 KINDS OF AI THAT ARE PERTINENT TO HEALTHCARE

A group of technologies collectively referred to as artificial intelligence. There is a significant range in the procedures and jobs they assist. The definition and description of some specific AI technologies that are extremely important to healthcare follow [10].

8.6.1 MACHINE LEARNING

A statistical technique called machine learning involves "teaching" models with data and "learning" by fitting models to that data. ML is the most widely used branch of AI; as mentioned by a Deloitte survey of 2018 involving 1,100 US managers, 63% of the businesses surveyed were utilizing ML. This general approach, on which many AI approaches are based, comes in a wide variety. The most important use of traditional ML in the healthcare sector is precision medicine that demonstrates the treatment techniques most likely to be effective on a patient, depending on a range of patient attributes. The most important application of ML and precision medicine is demanding supervised learning, which makes use of a training dataset with a known end variable (like the beginning of disease). Figure 8.4 shows the modeling machine learning in healthcare.

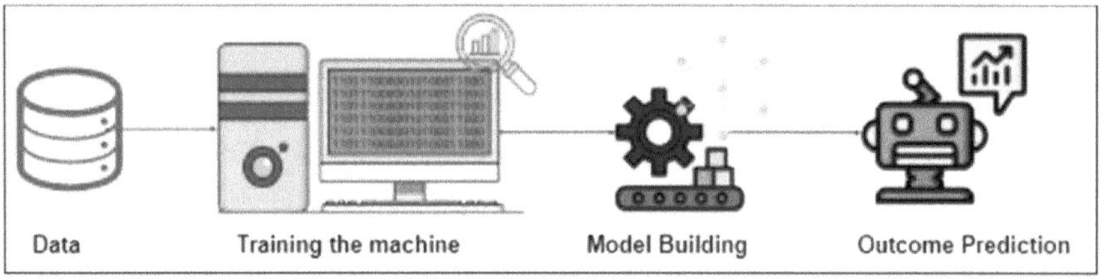

FIGURE 8.4 Modeling ML in healthcare for predicting outcomes.

8.6.2 DEEP LEARNING

Deep learning, which uses neural network models with several levels of features or variables to predict outcomes, is one of the more difficult types of machine learning. These models might have tens of thousands of hidden components that modern graphics processors and cloud computing platforms can handle more quickly. In the medical field, deep learning [12] is regularly used to spot potentially cancerous tumors in radiological images.

8.6.3 NEURAL NETWORKS

The neural network is a more advanced type of machine learning. This technology, which has been around since the 1960s and has been widely employed in medical research for several decades, is used for categorization tasks like predicting whether a patient would contract a specific disease. It approaches issues in terms of variables' weights, or "features," that link inputs and outputs [13]. It has been compared to how neurons interpret signals; however, the comparison to how the brain works is not very strong.

8.6.4 NATURAL LANGUAGE PROCESSING

Since the 1950s, researchers in AI have been striving to understand how human language works. NLP encompasses a variety of applications that deal with language, including speech recognition, text analysis, translation, and other tasks. The two main methods are statistical and semantic NLP. Statistical NLP is based on ML and specifically on deep learning neural networks, has recently enabled improvements in recognition accuracy. To learn a language, you need a sizable "corpus" or body of knowledge.

8.6.5 ROBOTIC PROCESS AUTOMATION

Information system administration duties that are organized are carried out by this technology as if being done by a human being. Instead of using physical robots, robotic process automation (RPA) usually uses server-based software [14]. It requires the integration of business rules, workflow, and presentation layer to perform as a sophisticated user of the information systems.

8.6.6 RULE-BASED SKILLED SYSTEMS

The matured systems relying on databases of "if-then" rules dominated artificial intelligence in the 1980s and the decades that followed. They have been widely utilized in the healthcare sector for "clinical decision support" in the last 20 years, and they are still widely utilized today [15]. Various electronic health record suppliers include a set of rules with their systems.

8.6.7 PHYSICAL ROBOTS

Physical robots are already well-known, with approximately 2,00,000 industrial robot installations occurring worldwide per year. They perform preset tasks including moving, lifting, welding, and assembling items in locations like factories and warehouses. Robots have become easier to instruct by having them carry out a desired task, which has enhanced their capacity to operate cooperatively with people [16]. Additionally, it would seem logical that as artificial intelligence develops across different fields, physical robots would eventually incorporate the same improvements in intelligence.

8.6.8 SURGICAL ROBOTS

Surgical robots give physicians "superpowers" by enhancing their vision, enabling them to make precise, noninvasive incisions, close wounds, and perform other surgical procedures. They were initially accepted in the USA in 2000. However, crucial decisions are still made by human surgeons. Head and neck surgery, prostate surgery, and gynecologic surgery are among the common surgical procedures performed with robotic surgery.

8.7 SCALING AI IN HEALTHCARE

The understanding of AI and its full potential in the field of medicine, particularly in terms of how it will impact personalized care, is still in its early stages. Respondents and survey participants have come to the conclusion that we should anticipate witnessing three phases of expanding AI in healthcare after considering the solutions now in place and the concepts in the pipeline [17].

- **Step I:** Solutions are first likely to concentrate on routine, repetitive, and primarily administrative procedures that take up a significant amount of time for doctors and nurses to optimize healthcare operations and increase adoption. In this initial phase, we would also include imaging-based AI tools, which are already in use in disciplines like ophthalmology, pathology, and radiology.
- **Step II:** We predict a growth in AI solutions, such as remote monitoring, AI-powered alerting systems, or virtual assistants that ease the transition from hospital-based to home-based care as patients take on increased responsibility for their own care in the second phase. In addition, NLP solutions may be utilized more frequently in healthcare facilities and at home during this phase, and AI may be used in more fields, such as neurology, cardiology, and oncology where advancements are already being made.
- **Step III:** We would anticipate seeing more AI solutions in clinical practice based on data from clinical trials in the third phase [18], as there is an increasing focus on improved and scaled clinical decision-support (CDS) tools in a sector that has learned from

prior attempts to introduce such tools into clinical practice and has modified its mindset, culture, and skills. In the end, respondents believed that AI would be fundamental to improving population health, learning, studying, and all other facets of the healthcare value chain. Figure 8.5 gives the list of AI applications for modernizing healthcare.

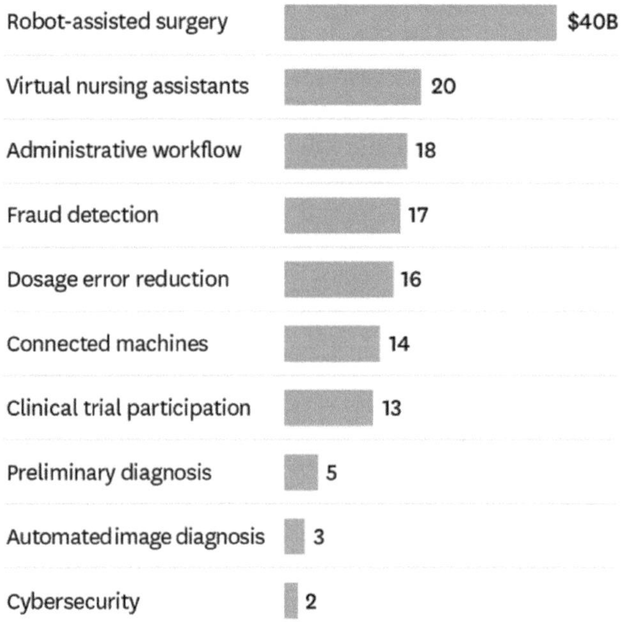

FIGURE 8.5 AI Applications for modernizing healthcare.

8.8 DIABETES PREDICATION – WITH THE USE OF ML

Data mining is becoming increasingly well-known and perhaps essential in the field of healthcare, with its highly focused and extensive uses in several associations [19]. Applications for data mining can greatly benefit every group involved in the medical services sector. It can be used by medical insurers to identify fraud and misuse, insurance organizations to decide how to manage client relationships, doctors to identify potent pharmaceuticals, and patients to obtain better and more affordable medical care. Data mining is a theory and technique that transforms enormous amounts of data into useful information for decision-making, which is a crucial component of managing medical services. Medical diagnosis is made feasible by methods and tools that can extract information from the vast amounts of data since medical services frameworks are both information-rich and knowledge-poor. Medical diagnosis is seen as a necessary but complex task that must be carried out precisely and successfully.

In India, diabetes is becoming a frequent condition. In India, there were approximately 31.7 million diabetic patients in 2000, and by 2030, there may be 79.4 million [20]. The mathematical methods known as machine learning algorithms are highly helpful for assessing vast amounts of data and making recommendations for actions based on that data. These formulas can be used to analyze a set of data and forecast the values of new entries. Numerous academics are using ML algorithms to predict and manage different diseases. The outcomes of machine learning algorithms were highly successful in predicting various diseases. Machine learning algorithms must be used to investigate their potential for predicting diabetes so that appropriate preventative measures can be adopted.

Diabetes is a chronic medical illness brought on by incorrect control of the body's glucose levels. It is the most common cause of death and a chronic condition that develops when blood glucose levels are too high. Planning a new strategy for diabetes prevention and management is essential as the disease's incidence rises [21]. The user convenience and accessibility of current disease management techniques, however, are limited. According to recent research, the creation of a disease management system with machine learning is an effective way to forecast the occurrence of diabetes in adults with high accuracy.

Diabetes is a chronic disorder marked by persistently elevated blood sugar or glucose levels in the sufferer [22]. Diabetes is generally characterized by an increase in thirst, hunger, weight loss, and frequent urination. People with diabetes run the danger of developing conditions including heart disease, neurological damage, etc. If early prediction is possible, the risk factor and seriousness of diabetes can be decreased. Machine learning plays a major role in the medical industry. By using several classification techniques, diabetes occurrence can be predicted (Random Forest and K-NN algorithms).

The most well-known kind of diabetes is type 2, which typically affects adults but is increasingly becoming a problem for children and teenagers. Since the body can produce insulin in this kind but it may not be enough or the body may not be able to respond to its effects, glucose continues to flow in the blood. This type is also known as insulin resistance. This category also includes LADA (Latent Autoimmune Diabetes in Adults), which describes a smaller proportion of people with type 2 diabetes who appear to have an impervious to loss of pancreatic beta cells [23]. Many people with type 2 diabetes can manage their blood sugar levels by adopting a balanced food plan and increasing their physical activity.

8.9 LITERATURE REVIEW

Sinha et al. [24] looked at a few AI applications, such as tele-diagnostics, robotic surgery, drug discovery, and cybersecurity that give medical personnel and systems additional anticipatory skills. Over the past few years, business models in the healthcare sector have changed. The costs and pricing of healthcare services will be the major area of change. The future of AI and digital technology in the healthcare sector was examined by authors. The future of healthcare must solve several important challenges. The chapter highlights significant analytics-related issues where cutting-edge methods like AI can play a significant role. It delves deeper into two key transformational areas: smart hospitals and the personal health cloud.

In their discussion of bias and justice in healthcare, Ahmad et al. [25] further discussed the potential for discrimination and the maintenance of unjust and prejudiced healthcare practices multiplies with the introduction of AI. The problems, needs, and opportunities in the field of fairness in healthcare AI, as well as the different intricacies related to it, are the main topics of focus. Various real-world examples are used to clarify the subject of healthcare as a multifaceted systems-level challenge that demands careful evaluation of various notions of fairness in healthcare to similar concepts in machine learning.

AI for social good (AI4SG) is a field of study that is focused on the idea that machine learning should be used for the good of society, as Monselise et al. [26] proved. We define AI4SG and concentrate on the most extensively researched application of AI4SG, healthcare, because the term's definition may be ambiguous or variable. Our study applies AI4SG principles to healthcare data that is either user-generated or obtained from electronic health records, and the results provide clinicians and the public with insightful information that can be used to address issues like vaccine misinformation, suicide prevention, and prostate cancer detection.

Future healthcare diagnostic tools and sensors will benefit from modern innovations and technology in heterogeneous integration technology, processes, materials, tools, and, according to Knickerbocker et al. [27]. AI systems provide information and recommendations to patients, healthcare providers, and the public with the hope of raising quality of life and reducing expenses. Examples include – (i) early detection of chronic diseases and the possibility of delaying or preventing disease progression; (ii) comprehension of individual behavior; (iii) personalized care relying on medical diagnostics, DNA, and healthcare trends that are related to your healthcare requirements and available methods for managing your quality of life.

With the goal of establishing accountability, transparency, result tracing, and model improvement in the healthcare industry, Pawar et al. [28] explored XAI as a technology that may be applied in the analysis and diagnosis of health data using AI-based systems. In the field of "explainable AI," methods are being developed to explain predictions produced by AI systems. To gather data regarding the various effective uses of AI in the healthcare industry, Kumar et al. [29] employed a case study technique. Since AI can undoubtedly serve as a useful complement to doctors in the future, its implications are urgently needed. This research will aid government officials, academics, and healthcare practitioners in creating solutions for social wellness. Through the effective application of AI, this study chapter will assist in advancing the healthcare industry. Since AI is the technology of the future and is always evolving, it requires rigorous research on a regular basis. Here, the goal is to become familiar with various AI applications in healthcare and to analyze how they may affect it, as they may have a substantial impact on the medical community.

Explainable AI (XAI), a disruptive trend in AI that focuses on the explicability of conventional AI models by utilizing the models' decision-making and prediction outputs, was explored by Saraswat et al. [30]. The explainability factor gives black-box models new potential and gives healthcare stakeholders the confidence to interpret ML and DL models. In the healthcare industry, transparency in predictive analysis is essential, and XAI is centered on enhancing clinical health practices. Recent studies on XAI in healthcare have not placed a substantial emphasis on data analysis and model interpretation, which reduces the likelihood of its practical application. Due to this lack, the proposed survey precisely describes the operational and data gathering process needs of XAI in Healthcare 5.0. The study proposes a proposed architecture for an XAI ensemble on the computed tomography (CT) image segmentation and classification process based on the review methodology and research topics that are addressed. The proposed solution taxonomy of XAI in Healthcare 5.0 is provided together with operational issues.

Han et al. [31] showed how the healthcare sector is a sizable industry with outdated systems that can cause inefficiencies. Governments and healthcare organizations have traditionally made the most of the investments, but now significant tech firms like Google and Microsoft are beginning to do so as well. Additionally, with the global COVID-19 outbreak, issues about digital healthcare are resurfacing. As new technologies develop and rules change because of pooled expertise, this has led to a significant movement in the areas of focus within the field of digital health. We shall examine the digital healthcare sector, its regulations, and its technological advancements in this essay.

The focus of this chapter will be on addressing the demands of the patient and clinicians without compromising, as Raj et al. [32] concentrated on doing. To solve this challenge, advanced computer systems, effective sensors, and IoT devices will all be crucial. This research necessitates extensive analysis, quick progress, and concurrent continuous research. This chapter offers information about research into the use of AI-based approaches in the healthcare industry for the benefit and convenience of medical professionals and patients. The introduction part covers fundamental concepts. To complete the research, we will use AI-based algorithms and cloud solutions.

Research on AI technology and its effects on the healthcare sector was given by Whig et al. [33]. According to the researchers' surveys, without AI technology, rapid progress in the healthcare sector would not be feasible. To save time and effort for focused work, it is crucial that all healthcare organizations employ AI technology. The study was conducted to determine whether artificial intelligence technology plays an important part in the UK healthcare industry.

Jahan et al. [34] developed a decentralized information capacity mechanism for a collaborative smart healthcare system that guarantees the interoperability and security of patient medical records. In the proposed approach, hospitals share patient data while ensuring data privacy via a differential privacy method in a decentralized database. The suggested system's viability is demonstrated by the analysis of experimental results and the accuracy of the data using an AI model.

With technological breakthroughs, businesses aspire to make revolutionary improvements to all parts of industries. The healthcare sector is struggling with a double load of sicknesses, a narrow scope of benefits, and a lack of a fundamental financial risk security system. Many healthcare companies still rely on regional centralized database systems to store patient health records. When patient information is stored in a hospital database, the integrity and privacy of that information are the major issues. Patient records that have been updated occasionally are not promptly placed in the database. Patients are also reluctant to provide their medical records due to privacy concerns. As a result, re-diagnosis is a laborious and costly process that raises the cost of healthcare.

Murray et al. [35] suggested an enhanced network of clinical notetaking, where coding is automatically created by an AI system when physicians write their clinical notes, as a solution to numerous problems. The technology (AI-KEN) provides improved web assistance that is connected to regional clinical systems, allowing clinical notes to be prompted by recommended predictive text possibilities in real time. The advantages envisioned include decreased financial loss for emergency services, assistance with maintaining healthcare standards, and improved real-time developments for clinical practice and research. This overcomes the problems relating to high expenses, a lack of data integration, and information loss that impacts the capacity to uphold standards in the delivery of clinical care and patient outcomes.

Sharma et al. [36] described how machine learning, algorithms, and software are used in healthcare to gather data, process it, and provide end users with a clear conclusion. Machine learning, deep learning, and algorithms are used by AI to do this. These algorithms develop their own logic after identifying a pattern in behavior. Analysis of the connections between the various treatment modalities is the main goal of health-related AI applications. A diagnostic procedure, medication research, tailored medicine, patient monitoring, and care all use AI-based tools. AI algorithms can also be used to analyze a lot of data and determine which patient health reports should come first, second, and third in order of importance. Authors describe the function and use of AI in smart healthcare systems. Sharma et al. [37] discussed the application of cutting-edge technologies like IoT, blockchain, and AI in telemedicine and smart healthcare. The three key IT-based cutting-edge technologies—AI, IoT, and Blockchain—are necessary at various stages of transforming traditional healthcare into smart healthcare.

Komal et al. [38] concentrated on the application of AI to mimic the capabilities and limitations of the human mind. By making healthcare and service information more accessible and hastening the development of investigative techniques, it is changing the way people think about constraints. Cardiology, cancer, and neurology are three significant disease areas where AI techniques are used. After reviewing the applications and ethical concerns in the use of AI in healthcare, we conclude regarding the various AI frameworks. To create trustworthy AI in the healthcare industry, Leung et al. [39] introduced an explainable AI (XAI) system that generates precise predictions and explains the forecasts. Results from evaluations using real-world datasets show how effective our XAI solution is for reliable AI in healthcare.

To build an intelligent therapeutic decision emotionally supportive network to aid the clinicians, Shetty et al. [40] focused on the medical conclusion learning design element using the diabetes data gathered. The major objective of this study is to develop an intelligent diabetes disease prediction system that examines the condition of diabetes using a database of diabetes patients. In this system, we propose analyzing a database of diabetes patients while utilizing algorithms like Bayesian and KNN (K-Nearest Neighbor) to analyze them while taking various diabetic attributes for diabetes sickness prediction.

Artificial neural network-based diabetes detection methods are evaluated by Paul et al. [41]. It includes a study on the scaled conjugate gradient backpropagation of ANN with k-fold cross-validation for the prediction of diabetic illness. Data from 768 diabetic patients, ranging in age from 21 to 81, is used to train the network. The quantity of neurons in the hidden layer determines how accurate the results are. The suggested system estimates the absence and presence of diabetes during testing, yielding a minimum accuracy percentage of 77% and a maximum accuracy percentage of 100%. It uses 8 input attributes. A multilayer perceptron neural network was used by Song et al. [42] to develop a diabetes incidence prediction system that allows users to enter basic data, enhancing predictability and convenience. The proposed approach performed well in terms of forecasting diabetes incidences when it was tested on Pima Indians.

A disease index grading approach based on the logistic regression algorithm was proposed by Lei et al. [43]. Based on the illness progression index score one year later, the findings are divided into two categories: greater than or equal to 150 and less than 150. The logistic regression model is a good fit for the challenge of determining which interval the goal value will belong to. The LR technique is a successful attempt to forecast the effect of a feature on the course of diabetes as opposed to utilizing this algorithm. The classification accuracy can be 75.7% when the two selected features are S5 and S6, according to the results of the logistic regression model.

A kernel-based adaptive filtering approach was put out by Sun et al. [44] to create prediction models for glucose prediction. Then, the specifics for choosing a suitable kernel function are also investigated. Lastly, the effectiveness of the suggested kernel-based forecasting approach is assessed in the prediction of short-term blood glucose levels. The performance of the suggested KLMS algorithm is further outlined through analysis of the relative outcomes. To maintain a normal blood glucose level, patients with type 1 diabetes (T1D) must undergo insulin injections. The development of a trustworthy prediction model is made possible by the continuous glucose monitoring (CGM) system's ability to regularly check the glucose level.

Support vector machine (SVM) was used in diabetes prediction by Mohan et al. [45]. The effectiveness of the SVM method is examined for the various kernels that are accessible. The most effective kernel is chosen and applied for prediction. Python is used to implement the suggested task, and its performance is on par with that of other algorithms. Han et al. [46] took into consideration the RapidMiner tool as a method for analyzing a Pima Indians Diabetes Data Set, which gathers patient information on those with and without getting diabetes, is based on its ability to analyze large data sets quickly. The discussion follows the data mining procedure. The emphasis will be on data preprocessing, which includes attribute selection and identification, numerical discretization, data normalization, outlier removal, the detection of hidden correlations, visual data analysis, and the development of a diabetes prediction model.

8.10 PROPOSED METHODOLOGY

A supervised learning used in this study is Random Forest classifier, an algorithm that performs classification and regression. It relies on the principle of merging multiple classifiers referred to as ensemble learning, often known as social learning. This is a technique employed to resolve complicated problems and enhance model performance.

It is made up of several tree-structured classifiers with the following structure: {h (x, V) n = 1, 2, ...}, where the {V} are independent, identically distributed random vectors, and each tree casts one unit of vote for the class that is most prevalent at input x. Random Forest Classifier creates a group of decision trees. The randomization strategy effectively achieves variation among base decision trees when used with bagging or the random subspace method. Each tree in Random Forest is created using a variety of steps: The bootstrap sample is used when there are N records in the training set and N records are picked at random but with replacement from the original data.

If there are K input variables, then $k << K$ is chosen such that k variables are randomly chosen from K at each node, and the best split on these k characteristics is used to split the node. Pruning is not done. The value of k is maintained constant during the growth of the forest (Figure 8.6).

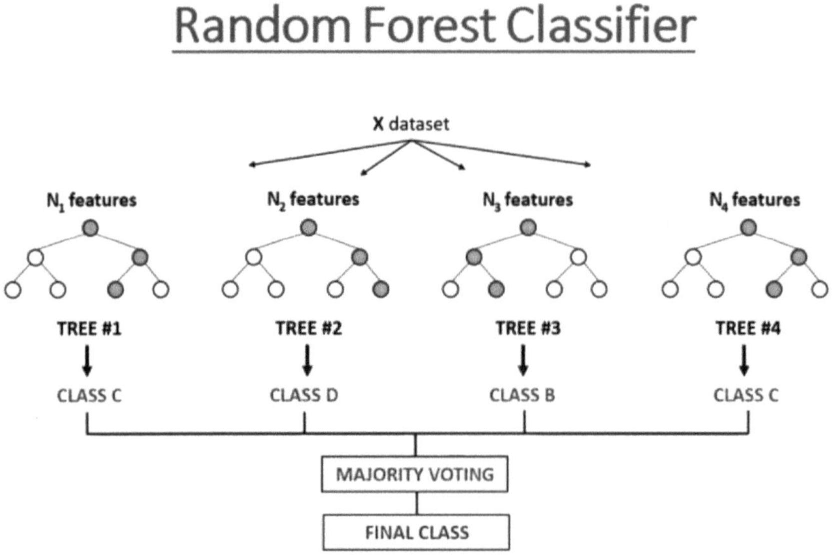

FIGURE 8.6 Random forest algorithm.

This results in a forest with many trees; the number of trees is predetermined by the parameter N. The node size parameter, which refers to the number of instances in the leaf node, can be used to determine the depth of the tree and is typically set to 1. Once the forest has been trained or constructed as described above, it is run across all the trees grown there to classify fresh instances. Each tree provides a classification, which is then recorded as a vote. After combining the votes from all trees, the class with the most votes (majority voting) is proclaimed as the classification of the new instance.

About one-third of the original instances are lost when the bootstrap sample set is created during the forest-building process by sampling with replacement for each tree. The OOB (Out-of-bag) data refers to this collection of instances. Errors are calculated using OOB error estimates, and each tree in the forest has its own OOB data set for this purpose. The built-in capabilities of the Random Forest method to calculate variable significance and proximities can be utilized to replace missing values and outliers.

The generalization error (PE*) of Random Forest is given as:

$$PE * = P\ x,\ y\ (mg\ (X,Y)) < 0$$

The margin function is mg(X, Y) that calculates how much the average vote for the correct class is more than the average vote for any other class. The classification is shown here, along with the predictor vector.

Figure 8.6 illustrates the working of the random forest classifier where each tree is given some N features. Based on these features, the tree is formed. Each tree provides its classification, and the classification class with the most votes is selected as the final output.

In Figure 8.7, the flowchart of the Random Forest algorithm with the diabetic dataset is explained. The diabetic dataset is collected from the PIDD. The dataset is pre-processed to handle any missing or invalid values. After preprocessing, a decision tree is formed using the training dataset. Once the training is completed, the dataset is tested with the training data set. The accuracy is evaluated by comparing the actual and target values.

The algorithm for random forest classifiers is as follows:

1. N represents the total number of cases in the training dataset, from which each case is randomly selected and replaced with data from the original dataset.
2. Individual decision trees are built for each sample, with predictors chosen randomly from input variables of size M at each node. The nodes are divided by the optimal split on the m predictors. The value of m remains constant during the growth of the forest.

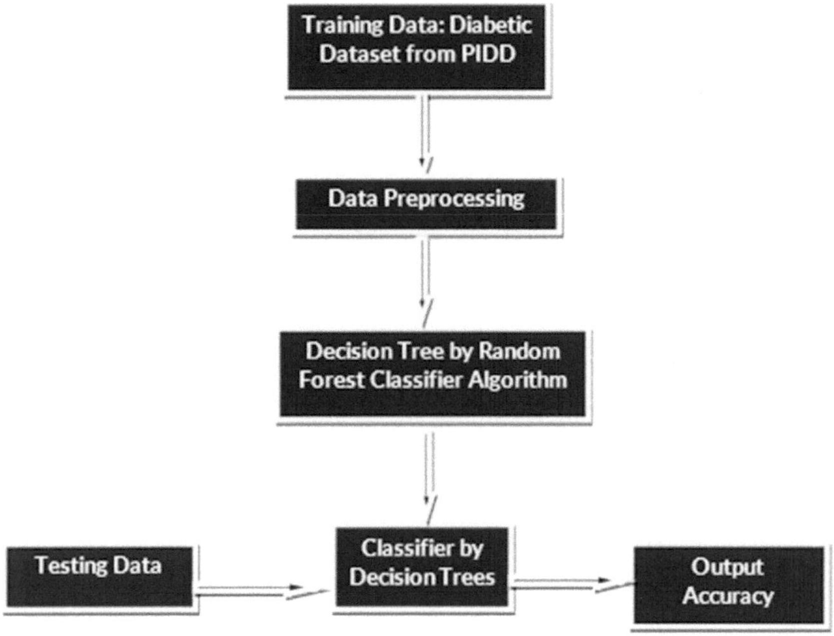

FIGURE 8.7 Flowchart for random forest algorithm.

3. The final output, which can be used for regression or classification, is determined by the majority vote or the average vote of all the decision trees.

The dataset is tested after the training phase to assess the correctness of the trained model. Approximately one-third of the cases in the training set are left out or subsided during sampling with replacement; these cases are known as Out-of-Bag (OOB) data. This OOB information is utilized to estimate classification errors for a test dataset.

8.10.1 DATASET DESCRIPTION

It is assumed that the dataset being used for analysis is representative of the nation's population and current healthcare costs. The National Institute of Diabetes and Digestive and Kidney Diseases of the NIH is the owner of the Pima Indian Diabetes Database (PIDD). The UC-Irvine Machine Learning Repository received it in 1990. Cross-checking is done on the dataset to look for any errors, excessive results, or discrepancies.

Title: Diabetes Database for Pima Indians
Instances: 768
Attributes: 8 (all values are numerical)

1. The number of pregnancies.
2. In an oral glucose tolerance test, the plasma glucose concentration after two hours.
3. Diastolic blood pressure (mm Hg).
4. The width of the triceps skin fold (mm).
5. Insulin 2-hour serum (mu U/ml).

   Body mass index is calculated as follows:

6. Diabetic family history.
7. Age (years).
8. Class variable 9 (1 or 0).

Missing Attribute Values: Yes
Class Distribution: (Class value 1 represents "tested positive for diabetes").

8.10.2 DATA ANALYSIS

Here, we're talking about the medical information related to diabetic individuals. There are two main categories in this collection of biomedical data. Table 8.1 depicts how these two major categories are distributed over the entire collection of data. People who do not have diabetes and those who do have the disease are the two categories.

TABLE 8.1 Class Distribution of Dataset

Class Value	Number of Instances
0	499
1	269

8.10.3 EXPERIMENTAL ANALYSIS AND RESULTS

The results are based on the accuracy achieved after applying random forest classifier on our dataset. In Figure 8.8, the class distribution of data is shown where 0 represents the number of non-diabetic patients, whereas the number 1 represents the diabetic patients with value counts of 500 and 268, respectively.

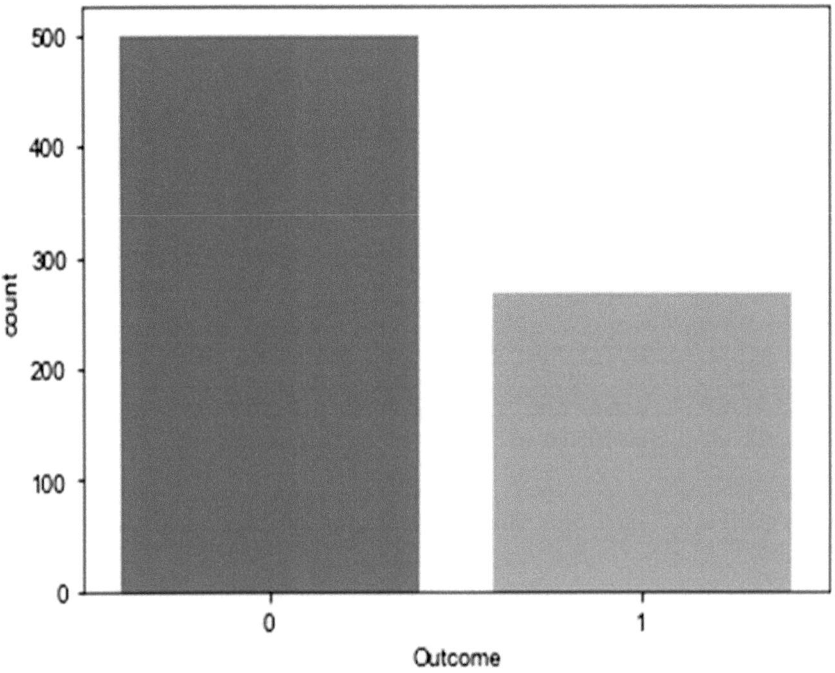

FIGURE 8.8 Class distribution of data.

For each parameter, we conduct the usual analysis on the dataset, which displays statistical indicators like the mean, minimum, and maximum values, standard deviation, and quantiles. The computed values for each indication are displayed in Figure 8.9.

	count	mean	std	min	25%	50%	75%	max
Pregnancies	768.0	3.845052	3.369578	0.000	1.00000	3.0000	6.00000	17.00
Glucose	768.0	120.894531	31.972618	0.000	99.00000	117.0000	140.25000	199.00
BloodPressure	768.0	69.105469	19.355807	0.000	62.00000	72.0000	80.00000	122.00
SkinThickness	768.0	20.536458	15.952218	0.000	0.00000	23.0000	32.00000	99.00
Insulin	768.0	79.799479	115.244002	0.000	0.00000	30.5000	127.25000	846.00
BMI	768.0	31.992578	7.884160	0.000	27.30000	32.0000	36.60000	67.10
iabetesPedigreeFunction	768.0	0.471876	0.331329	0.078	0.24375	0.3725	0.62625	2.42
Age	768.0	33.240885	11.760232	21.000	24.00000	29.0000	41.00000	81.00
Outcome	768.0	0.348958	0.476951	0.000	0.00000	0.0000	1.00000	1.00

FIGURE 8.9 Characters and statistical indicators of dataset.

Here Figure 8.10 shows the classification report of RF in terms of recall, precision, F1-Score, and support values.

	precision	recall	f1-score	support
0	1.00	1.00	1.00	151
1	1.00	1.00	1.00	80
accuracy			1.00	231
macro avg	1.00	1.00	1.00	231
weighted avg	1.00	1.00	1.00	231

FIGURE 8.10 Classification report for RFC.

In Figure 8.11, Confusion matrix shows the four values which is true positive, false positive true negative, and false negative.

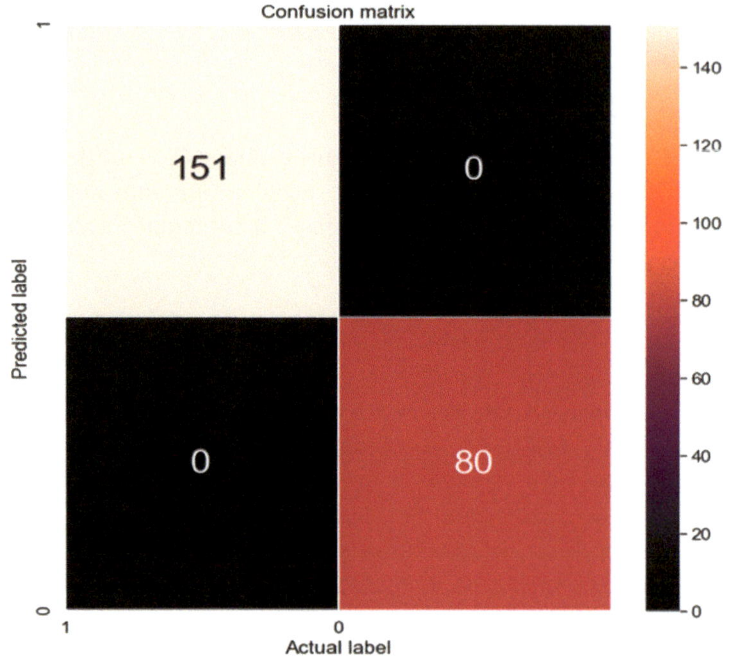

FIGURE 8.11 Confusion matrix for RFC.

8.11 CONCLUSION

Machine learning and other cognitive sciences are used in healthcare AI to make medical diagnoses. AI is improving in performing human-like tasks more quickly, efficiently, and affordably. Robotics and artificial intelligence have a lot of potential in healthcare. Medical machine learning algorithms can be applied to the assessment of critical clinical parameters, predictions of various diseases, predicting pharmacological assignments, extraction of medical knowledge, support for treatment planning, and patient management. Various algorithms of machine learning and deep learning can be used for prediction and analysis in the field of the healthcare industry. When the individual supplies the value of the necessary characteristic, the Random Forest classifier has been employed in this chapter with various test parameters, and it has been discovered that it is useful in the diagnosis of Diabetes mellitus. The confusion matrix and classification report of the results are shown. We may conclude from an analysis of the confusion matrix that the accuracy of our Random Forest Classifier-based technique is superior. Hybrid classification techniques may be used in future research to improve the suggested system's overall performance.

KEYWORDS

- **artificial intelligence**
- **deep learning**
- **diabetes mellitus**
- **diabetes prediction**
- **healthcare**
- **hybrid classification techniques**
- **machine learning**
- **random forest classifier**

REFERENCES

1. Guo, Y., Hao, Z., Zhao, S., Gong, J., & Yang, F. (2020). Artificial intelligence in health care: Bibliometric analysis. *Journal of Medical Internet Research, 22*(7), e18228. https://doi.org/10.2196/18228.
2. Choudhury, A., Renjilian, E., & Asan, O. (2020). Use of machine learning in geriatric clinical care for chronic diseases: A systematic literature review. *JAMIA Open, 3*(3), 459–471. https://doi.org/10.1093/jamiaopen/ooaa025.
3. Tran, B. X., Vu, G. T., Ha, G. H., Vuong, Q. H., Ho, M. T., Vuong, T. T., et al. (2019). Global evolution of research in artificial intelligence in health and medicine: A bibliometric study. *Journal of Clinical Medicine, 8*(3), 360. https://doi.org/10.3390/jcm8030360.
4. Tagliaferri, S. D., Angelova, M., Zhao, X., Owen, P. J., Miller, C. T., Wilkin, T., et al. (2020). Artificial intelligence to improve back pain outcomes and lessons learnt from clinical classification approaches: Three systematic reviews. *NPJ Digital Medicine, 3*(1), 1–16. https://doi.org/10.1038/s41746-020-0252-7.
5. Shortliffe, E. H., & Sepúlveda, M. J. (2018). Clinical decision support in the era of artificial intelligence. *JAMA, 320*(21), 2199–2200. https://doi.org/10.1001/jama.2018.17163.
6. Dos Santos, B. S., Steiner, M. T. A., Fenerich, A. T., & Lima, R. H. P. (2019). Data mining and machine learning techniques applied to public health problems: A bibliometric analysis from 2009 to 2018. *Computers & Industrial Engineering, 138*, 106120. https://doi.org/10.1016/j.cie.2019.106120.
7. Panch, T., Szolovits, P., & Atun, R. (2018). Artificial intelligence, machine learning and health systems. *Journal of Global Health, 8*(2), 020303. https://doi.org/10.7189/jogh.08.020303.
8. Liao, H., Tang, M., Luo, L., Li, C., Chiclana, F., & Zeng, X.-J. (2018). A bibliometric analysis and visualization of medical big data research. *Sustainability, 10*(1), 166. https://doi.org/10.3390/su10010166.
9. Mach, M. A., & Abdel-Badeeh, M. S. (2010). Intelligent techniques for business intelligence in healthcare. In *2010 10th International Conference on Intelligent Systems Design and Applications* (pp. 545–550). https://doi.org/10.1109/ISDA.2010.5687145.
10. Ramakrishnan, N., Hanauer, D., & Keller, B. (2010). Mining electronic health records. *Computer, 43*(10), 77–81. https://doi.org/10.1109/MC.2010.309.
11. Kulkarni, P., Mahabaleshwarkar, A., Kulkarni, M., Sirsikar, N., & Gadgil, K. (2019). Conversational AI: An overview of methodologies, applications & future scope. In *2019 5th International Conference on Computing, Communication, Control and Automation (ICCUBEA)* (pp. 1–7). https://doi.org/10.1109/ICCUBEA47591.2019.9128834.
12. Chan, H.-C., Chen, J.-C., Chien, S.-W., Chen, Y.-F., & Bau, C.-T. (2012). Evaluation of intelligent system to the control of diabetes. In *2012 International Symposium on Computer, Consumer and Control* (pp. 585–588). https://doi.org/10.1109/IS3C.2012.165.

13. Kalis, B., Collier, M., & Fu, R. (2018, May 10). 10 promising AI applications in health care. *Harvard Business Review*. https://hbr.org/2018/05/10-promising-ai-applications-in-health-care (accessed on 31 May 2024).
14. Wallace, E., & Smith, S. M., & Fahey, T. (2012). Variation in medical practice: Getting the balance right. *Family Practice, 29*(5), 501–502. https://doi.org/10.1093/fampra/cmr103.
15. Balicer, R. D., & Cohen-Stavi, C. (2020). Advancing healthcare through data-driven medicine and artificial intelligence. In B. Nordlinger, C. Villani, & D. Rus (Eds.), *Healthcare and Artificial Intelligence*. Springer, Cham. https://doi.org/10.1007/978-3-030-36987-3_8.
16. Belciug, S. (2022). A statistical analysis handbook for validating artificial intelligence techniques applied in healthcare. In C. P. Lim, Y. W. Chen, A. Vaidya, C. Mahorkar, & L. C. Jain (Eds.), *Handbook of Artificial Intelligence in Healthcare* (Intelligent Systems Reference Library, Vol. 212). Springer, Cham. https://doi.org/10.1007/978-3-030-72892-2_2.
17. Triberti, S., Durosini, I., La Torre, D., Sebri, V., Savioni, L., & Pravettoni, G. (2022). Artificial intelligence in healthcare practice: How to tackle the "human" challenge. In C. P. Lim, Y. W. Chen, A. Vaidya, C. Mahorkar, & L. C. Jain (Eds.), *Handbook of Artificial Intelligence in Healthcare* (Intelligent Systems Reference Library, Vol. 212). Springer, Cham. https://doi.org/10.1007/978-3-030-72892-2_3.
18. Albu, A., Precup, R. E., & Teban, T. A. (2022). Intelligent paradigms for diagnosis, prediction and control in healthcare applications. In C. P. Lim, Y. W. Chen, A. Vaidya, C. Mahorkar, & L. C. Jain (Eds.), *Handbook of Artificial Intelligence in Healthcare* (Intelligent Systems Reference Library, Vol. 212). Springer, Cham. https://doi.org/10.1007/978-3-030-72892-2_4.
19. Sun, X., Yu, X., Liu, J., & Wang, H. (2017). Glucose prediction for type 1 diabetes using KLMS algorithm. In *2017 36th Chinese Control Conference (CCC)* (pp. 1124–1128). https://doi.org/10.23919/ChiCC.2017.8027424.
20. Mohan, N., & Jain, V. (2020). Performance analysis of support vector machine in diabetes prediction. In *2020 4th International Conference on Electronics, Communication and Aerospace Technology (ICECA)* (pp. 1–3). https://doi.org/10.1109/ICECA49313.2020.9297483.
21. Han, J., Rodriguez, J. C., & Beheshti, M. (2008). Diabetes data analysis and prediction model discovery using RapidMiner. In *2008 Second International Conference on Future Generation Communication and Networking* (pp. 96–99). https://doi.org/10.1109/FGCN.2008.77.
22. VijiyaKumar, K., Lavanya, B., Nirmala, I., & Caroline, S. S. (2019). Random forest algorithm for the prediction of diabetes. In *2019 IEEE International Conference on System, Computation, Automation and Networking (ICSCAN)* (pp. 1–5). https://doi.org/10.1109/ICSCAN.2019.8878861.
23. Purushottam, Saxena, K., & Sharma, R. (2015). Diabetes mellitus prediction system evaluation using C4.5 rules and partial tree. In *2015 4th International Conference on Reliability, Infocom Technologies and Optimization (ICRITO) (Trends and Future Directions)* (pp. 1–6). https://doi.org/10.1109/ICRITO.2015.7359276.
24. Sinha, S., & Al Huraimel, K. (2021). Transforming healthcare with AI. In *Reimagining Businesses with AI* (pp. 33–54). Wiley. https://doi.org/10.1002/9781119642192.ch3.

25. Ahmad, M. A., Eckert, C., Allen, C., Kumar, V., Hu, J., & Teredesai, A. (2021). Fairness in healthcare AI. In *2021 IEEE 9th International Conference on Healthcare Informatics (ICHI)* (pp. 554–555). https://doi.org/10.1109/ICHI52183.2021.00103.
26. Monselise, M., & Yang, C. C. (2022). AI for social good in healthcare: Moving towards a clear framework and evaluating applications. In *2022 IEEE 10th International Conference on Healthcare Informatics (ICHI)* (pp. 470–471). https://doi.org/10.1109/ICHI54592.2022.00123.
27. Knickerbocker, J. U., et al. (2018). Heterogeneous integration technology demonstrations for future healthcare, IoT, and AI computing solutions. In *2018 IEEE 68th Electronic Components and Technology Conference (ECTC)* (pp. 1519–1528). https://doi.org/10.1109/ECTC.2018.00231.
28. Pawar, U., O'Shea, D., Rea, S., & O'Reilly, R. (2020). Explainable AI in healthcare. In *2020 International Conference on Cyber Situational Awareness, Data Analytics and Assessment (CyberSA)* (pp. 1–2). https://doi.org/10.1109/CyberSA49311.2020.9139678.
29. Kumar, A., & Joshi, S. (2022). Applications of AI in healthcare sector for enhancement of medical decision making and quality of service. In *2022 International Conference on Decision Aid Sciences and Applications (DASA)* (pp. 37–41). https://doi.org/10.1109/DASA54658.2022.9891724.
30. Saraswat, D., et al. (2022). Explainable AI for Healthcare 5.0: Opportunities and challenges. *IEEE Access, 10*, 84486–84517. https://doi.org/10.1109/ACCESS.2022.3195542.
31. Han, J. H., & Lee, J. Y. (2021). Digital healthcare industry and technology trends. In *2021 IEEE International Conference on Big Data and Smart Computing (BigComp)* (pp. 375–377). https://doi.org/10.1109/BigComp51126.2021.00070.
32. Raj, S. D., & Karthiban. (2022). Applications of artificial intelligence in healthcare. In *2022 International Conference on Computer Communication and Informatics (ICCCI)* (pp. 1–2). https://doi.org/10.1109/ICCCI54379.2022.9740875.
33. Whig, V., Othman, B., Haque, M. A., Gehlot, A., Qamar, S., & Singh, J. (2022). An empirical analysis of artificial intelligence (AI) as a growth engine for the healthcare sector. In *2022 2nd International Conference on Advance Computing and Innovative Technologies in Engineering (ICACITE)* (pp. 2454–2457). https://doi.org/10.1109/ICACITE53722.2022.9823772.
34. Jahan, N., Rashid, I. B., Al Numan, O., Hasan, A. S. M. T., & Begum, N. (2021). Collaborative AI in smart healthcare system. In *2021 International Conference on Automation, Control and Mechatronics for Industry 4.0 (ACMI)* (pp. 1–5). https://doi.org/10.1109/ACMI53878.2021.9528244.
35. Murray, M., Macedo, M., & Glynn, C. (2019). Delivering health intelligence for healthcare services. In *2019 First International Conference on Digital Data Processing (DDP)* (pp. 88–91). https://doi.org/10.1109/DDP.2019.00021.
36. Sharma, H. K., Kumar, A., Pant, S., & Ram, M. (2022). Application of artificial intelligence in smart healthcare. In *Artificial Intelligence, Blockchain and IoT for Smart Healthcare* (pp. 37–46). River Publishers. https://doi.org/10.13052/rp9788770227077.ch3.
37. Sharma, H. K., Kumar, A., Pant, S., & Ram, M. (2022). Role of artificial intelligence, IoT and blockchain in smart healthcare. In *Artificial Intelligence, Blockchain and*

IoT for Smart Healthcare (pp. 25–36). River Publishers. https://doi.org/10.13052/rp9788770227077.ch2.

38. Komal, Sethi, G. K., Ahmad, N., Rehman, M. B., Dafallaa, H. M. E. I., & Rashid, M. (2021). Use of artificial intelligence in healthcare systems: State-of-the-art survey. In *2021 2nd International Conference on Intelligent Engineering and Management (ICIEM)* (pp. 243–248). https://doi.org/10.1109/ICIEM51511.2021.9445384.
39. Leung, C. K., Madill, E. W. R., Souza, J., & Zhang, C. Y. (2022). Towards trustworthy artificial intelligence in healthcare. In *2022 IEEE 10th International Conference on Healthcare Informatics (ICHI)* (pp. 626–632). https://doi.org/10.1109/ICHI54592.2022.00118.
40. Shetty, D., Rit, K., Shaikh, S., & Patil, N. (2017). Diabetes disease prediction using data mining. In *2017 International Conference on Innovations in Information, Embedded and Communication Systems (ICIIECS)* (pp. 1–5). https://doi.org/10.1109/ICIIECS.2017.8276012.
41. Paul, B., & Karn, B. (2021). Diabetes mellitus prediction using hybrid artificial neural network. In *2021 IEEE Bombay Section Signature Conference (IBSSC)* (pp. 1–5). https://doi.org/10.1109/IBSSC53089.2021.9662056.
42. Song, H., & Lee, S. (2021). Implementation of diabetes incidence prediction using a multilayer perceptron neural network. In *2021 IEEE International Conference on Bioinformatics and Biomedicine (BIBM)* (pp. 3089–3091). https://doi.org/10.1109/BIBM52615.2021.9669698.
43. Lei, L. (2020). Prediction of score of diabetes progression index based on logistic regression algorithm. In *2020 International Conference on Virtual Reality and Intelligent Systems (ICVRIS)* (pp. 954–956). https://doi.org/10.1109/ICVRIS51149.2020.00198.
44. Sun, X., Yu, X., Liu, J., & Wang, H. (2017). Glucose prediction for type 1 diabetes using KLMS algorithm. In *2017 36th Chinese Control Conference (CCC)* (pp. 1124–1128). https://doi.org/10.23919/ChiCC.2017.8027471.
45. Han, J., Rodriguez, J. C., & Beheshti, M. (2008). Diabetes data analysis and prediction model discovery using RapidMiner. In *2008 Second International Conference on Future Generation Communication and Networking* (pp. 96–99). https://doi.org/10.1109/FGCN.2008.77.
46. Kumar, K. V., Lavanya, B., Nirmala, I., & Caroline, S. S. (2019). Random forest algorithm for the prediction of diabetes. In *2019 IEEE International Conference on System, Computation, Automation and Networking (ICSCAN)* (pp. 1–5). https://doi.org/10.1109/ICSCAN.2019.8878861.

CHAPTER 9

A Survey on Artificial Intelligence and Machine Learning Approaches for Medical Data Authentication

B. MADHUSHREE,[1] A. V. SENTHIL KUMAR,[2] and H. R. CHENNAMMA[3]

[1]*JSS Science and Technology University, Mysore, Karnataka, India*

[2]*Hindusthan College of Arts and Science, Coimbatore, Tamil Nadu, India*

[3]*JSS Science and Technology University, Mysore, Karnataka, India*

ABSTRACT

Most medical image interpretations are traditionally handled by radiologists and doctors. But recently, researchers and medical professionals have started to utilize computer-assisted interventions due to significant pathological diversity and potential expert weariness. While computerized medical image analysis is lagging behind other medical imaging technologies in terms of advancements, it has been lately improved by machine learning (ML) and deep learning (DL) methods. ML and DL methods help to train the model and extract the features. On the other hand, the impact of advancements in medical imaging technologies on authentication of medical data is also significant. Since it is required to maintain confidentiality, medical data authentication is very much essential. This survey presents recent advancements in medical imaging with respect to artificial intelligence and the purposes of authentication in different fields.

Data-Driven Analytics for Healthcare: Artificial Intelligence and Machine Learning for Medical Diagnostics. Meghna Sharma, Priyanka Vashisht, A. V. Senthil Kumar, Chitra Singh, and Abdelmalek Amine (Eds.)

9.1 INTRODUCTION

Due to the global expansion of multimedia information and better Internet technology, users have simple access methods for storing, copying, and disseminating digital data for a variety of potential uses. Providing security and copyright protection for computerized content is a difficult task at the current time. Furthermore, there has been an increase in cyber-crime overall, as well as escalating offenses like fraud, illicit copying and information dissemination, and privacy leaks. Many applications require security to protect their data from unauthorized access (*refer to* Figure 9.1). Among these, medical science is a crucial field that deals with the analysis of human health data. Modern medical science has made significant strides in the field of medical imaging, which is crucial in the therapy of many disorders. These medical images are also referred to as diagnostic images and are classified into different forms, including radiography, tomography, dental radiography, colonoscopy, mammography, ultrasound, and magnetic resonance imaging, among others. Numerous patient medical data photographs are stored in hospital systems due to their extensive use in diagnostic treatments. This poses problems with data management and security. Attackers can readily modify the diagnostic data when it is transferred over an open transmission network, which can result in major problems related to incorrect treatment and diagnosis. Therefore, it is important that medical science addresses these two issues that are connected to diagnostic imaging. The authentication has various notable applications as shown in Figure 9.1. Currently, it is utilized for broadcast monitoring, assisting the content owner to keep an eye on the distribution of their work across numerous channels. It is commonly used in medical applications for authenticating and transmitting highly private patient information. Implementing this method in the electronic voting system can greatly minimize security maintenance required when conducting elections. In the case of companies for login details, biometrics are used, and in the case of renewal and claiming of licenses and insurance, authentication is much required.

The prominent form of medical data is in image format. Authentication of such images has many applications. In this survey, we have mentioned three purposes as shown in Figure 9.2. They are authentication for tampering detection, authentication for tampering localization, and authentication for recovery of data. The purpose of authentication in tampering detection

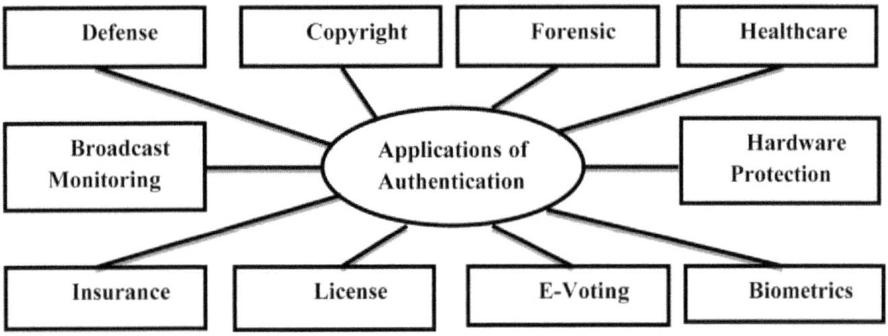

FIGURE 9.1 Application of authentication.

means the hash value will be generated for the whole image or with respect to the region of interest (ROI). At the receiving end, the user is going to check with the hash value. If it is different, then we claim it as a tampered image. Similarly, in the case of tampering localization, a hash value will be generated for each block of the image. If anything is modified, then check with the hash value of each block and localize the tampered area. At the same time, recovery of data can be generated using pixel values of ROI. By employing ROI pixel values, it may guarantee a recovery of the tampered area. This will increase the payload, and still, certain techniques lack to recover that much data.

In this dynamic field of medical imaging research, machine learning and deep learning techniques are quickly expanding. A lot of work is being done to improve medical applications using these machine and deep learning algorithms to detect flaws in diagnostic systems that could lead to incredibly unclear medical treatments. These techniques help to train the system to make better predictions and decision-making. The subject of ML makes computers master without being expressly programmed. Figure 9.2 shows the Classification of authentication.

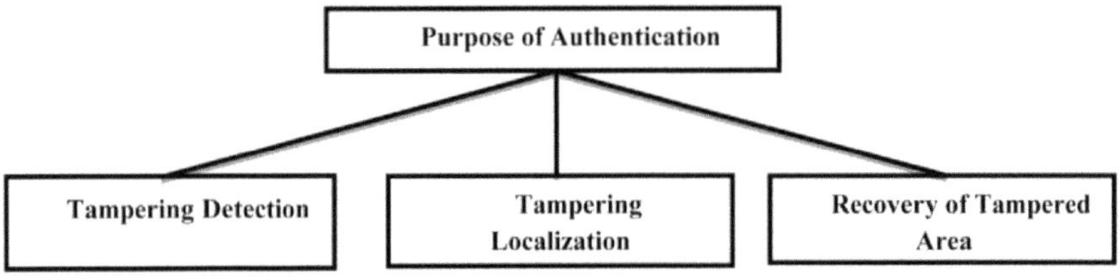

FIGURE 9.2 Classification of authentication purposes.

Deep learning is a type of machine learning that enables systems to understand the world in terms of reality with respect to a chain of thoughts. This domain provides insight into a computer where it can extract exact patterns from the given data and then process them for automatic reasoning. The fast-expanding field of medical imaging is used to detect diseases early and treat them. The role of image processing in the healthcare field is to connect with the expanding use of medical imaging. According to certain estimates, digital image processing has a significant impact on the decision-making process because it provides more accurate feature extraction. The methods of digital image processing are integrated into a wide range of computer systems. Due to advancements in image processing, authentication of medical images is essential and has an impact on system performance. As a result, it influences decisions and behaviors depending on methods in medical imaging. It provides numerous basic and sophisticated imaging techniques and visualization techniques [1]. DL and ML are major domains within artificial intelligence [2]. Artificial intelligence (AI) is the main field used to demonstrate human intellect in a machine. Machine learning is used to create AI, while deep learning is a technology used to apply machine learning. Before the output is detected, several stages are carried out on medical pictures. First, the machine and deep learning algorithms take the medical image as input. The image is then broken into many segments, and the desired location is zoomed in. Then noise is eliminated after choosing the desired features. The extracted data is then classified by the classifier, and predictions will be made based on this categorization. Every machine learning experiment follows these steps. The primary types of machine learning include supervised, semi-supervised, unsupervised, reinforcement, and active learning algorithms. Additionally, deep learning techniques are essentially an improved version of machine learning algorithms that use neural networks to classify data and make predictions with greater accuracy [3, 4].

Artificial intelligence is sub-categorized into two domains that includes:

- Machine learning;
- Deep learning.

9.1.1 MACHINE LEARNING

Medical science is a crucial field that deals with the analysis of human health data. Modern science in medicine has made significant strides in medical imaging, which is crucial in the diagnosis of many disorders. Numerous patient data are stored in hospital systems due to the extensive use of diagnostic images in treatments, which pose problems with data management and security. Attackers can easily modify diagnostic data when it is transferred over an insecure network, which further contributes to major problems with incorrect treatment and diagnosis. In medical image processing, various types of items, such as lesions and organs, can be too complex to be accurately depicted by a straightforward mathematical solution [5]. The author describes how they examined medical photos for disorders using pixel-based analysis. Medical image processing introduced pixel analysis in machine learning, which employs specific values in images directly as input data rather than features extracted from chunks. For some issues, the implementation of this technique may be superior to that of straightforward feature-based classifiers. Investigating the qualities of an image with poor variance is a challenging problem. In pixel-based machine learning algorithms, feature calculation and segmentation are not necessary, unlike conventional classifiers that aim to avoid errors caused by incorrect segmentation and feature generation. Due to the high dimensionality of the input, extensive training is required for pixel analysis. In Ref. [6], Agarwal et al. focused on analyzing low-quality diagnostic images. They utilized an efficient histogram equalization technique to enhance the image quality. This involved a two-part processing procedure, with the first phase enhancing global contrast through histogram adjustment. Additionally, homographic filtering was used for image sharpening. Fu et al. proposed a subsampling-based watermarking technique [7], where DWT was applied to obtain coefficients for sub-images derived from the original image. Support vector regression was then applied to each sub-image, and watermarks were embedded in the low-frequency coefficients. This algorithm demonstrated good performance against attacks. A novel approach based on support vector machines was introduced to address issues related to attacks [8]. This algorithm proves to be more robust against various attacks compared to other algorithms [5–7]. Here, a multiwavelet domain is used to employ a watermarking algorithm. At the first level, a single multiwavelet is applied to decompose each block of the image, and then mean modulation is applied. This modulation modulates the mean value and coefficients in two approximate sub-bands. These sub-bands are used to embed the watermark. Finally, a support vector machine (SVM) is applied to the watermarking image due to its high learning capability. This SVM extracts the watermark correctly under different attacks. Authentication for color medical images also plays an important role in the present situation. Sun et al. proposed a blind watermarking method for color medical images using PCA [9]. In this chapter, the authors applied the K-L transform to the medical image, and a binary watermark is embedded in the low-frequency sub-band of DWT. Then, the Human Visual System (HVS) is used to decide the block to embed the watermark, and the watermarked image is constructed. Ramly et al. proposed a new method to embed a watermark on medical images using SVM and spread spectrum [10]. There are three stages to secure medical images: first is to classify an image into Region of Interest (ROI) and Region of Non-Interest (RONI), then embed the patient data into the image, and lastly extract the data from the watermarked image. Here, at the stage of embedding, image-specific techniques should be used to enhance performance. Among all techniques, SVM is used because of its excellence in classification, and this SVM boosts the performance of the watermarking. Then, spread spectrum is used in the embedding stage because of its robustness to geometric attacks and to avoid degradation of image quality. To avoid manipulation of medical data on a public network, Rathi proposed a detailed analysis of watermarking based on medical images [11]. The author has provided a detailed study about medical image watermarking and the different domains used to embed the watermark. When it comes to medical image watermarking, embedding information and the type of image also play an important role. To provide security for healthcare data, Alamgir et al. presented a fuzzy clustering watermark [12]. First, the original image is segmented into three different classes including gray matter, cerebrospinal fluid, and white matter using fuzzy c-means. The gray matter is taken as concealing watermark and is divided into 8*8 blocks to calculate the entropy, contrast, and energy. This information is then given as input to the fuzzy c-means (FCM). Suitable blocks are extracted from FCM to embed the watermark. For the selected block, DCT and DWT are applied to extract the transformed block, and finally, the Arnold transform is applied to obtain the watermark. Ownership identification is a tedious task in the present situation. Emami proposed ownership identification for medical images using SVM and Lagrange duality [13]. To identify the ownership of electronic patient record (EPR) data, the author proposed this technique, which is categorized into two independent classes. One is to detect the watermarked image, and the other is to detect the non-watermarked image. Here BiLSB is used to classify between watermarked and non-watermarked. This algorithm decreases false positive and false negative errors. Watermarking is increasing day by day to enhance security, integrity, and confidentiality. However, watermarking for medical images is a special category in watermarking. Hence, DWT is applied to the original image for embedding the data. For extraction, independent component analysis is used. Finally, the quality of watermark embedding, and extraction is calculated in terms of Normalized Correlation (NC) and Peak Signal to Noise Ratio (PSNR) values [14]. An efficient algorithm is presented for integrity control in medical images [15]. Here, the medical image is divided into ROI and RONI parts. Firstly, the ROI part is taken, then the hash value for ROI is computed and named H1. Furthermore, ROI is divided into 'n' number of blocks. Then, for each block, hash value and geometric moments are calculated, resulting in H2 and H3. Finally, the ROI block is embedded with H1, H2, H3, and RONI as a watermark. The performance of this algorithm is improved compared to other embedding algorithms. Reversible watermarking retrieves the image and message perfectly, so Nguyen proposed this technique for medical images [16]. Firstly, the image is divided into a cross set and a dot set to generate an encrypted watermark. Secondly, embed the watermark at the LSB of 51 of each block. Then PSNR values are calculated to check the imperceptibility of the proposed algorithm by comparing it with other algorithms. To maintain medical image quality and to recover the tampered area, Badshah presented a lossless compression method using Lempel-Ziv-Welch (LZW) [17]. The watermark is created as a combination of the ROI part and a secret key. This watermark is then converted into binary format, compressed using LZW, and embedded into the original image. The watermarked image is then transmitted over a channel. At the receiving end, the user extracts the original image and watermark.

Tele-medicine is an application that transfers medical data from one hospital to another, making authentication of medical data important. Here, the input image is divided into 4×4 non-overlapping blocks. For each block, SVD is applied to calculate the median value. Then a master key is generated for the input image. On the other hand, the patient ID is encrypted using the Arnold cat map for the original image. Finally, this master key and patient ID are embedded into the medical image for double authentication purposes [18]. Suganya focuses on authenticating the medical image with respect to tamper detection [19]. This authentication is based on fragile watermarking technique. The original image is divided into m*n blocks and then converted into 8-bit planes. Then, at each least significant bit of the plane, K-means is applied. Next, clusters will be formed based on the K-means algorithm. The cluster values are used as a secret key to embed within the medical image. To increase robustness, Dhavale proposed a scheme where a barcode is embedded as a watermark to authenticate the medical image [20]. To generate the barcode, the patient ID is taken and then converted into a barcode image format. On the other hand, the original image is divided into 8*8 blocks and DCT is applied to each block. Then these blocks are given as input to K-means clustering. This clustering is divided into two clusters: one is HEBs and the other one is LEBs based on the energy values. Next, DCT blocks are randomly selected and quantized using a quality factor. After quantization, the image is ready for embedding the watermark. If the block is marked as HEB, then 4 bits of watermark information can be embedded. This algorithm is robust to compression attacks.

To avoid modification in the diagnosis part of the image, Rai et al. proposed an SVM-based watermarking technique [21]. This scheme provides double protection by embedding the watermark into the medical image. Firstly, the watermark is generated by producing a unique key, then it is embedded into the host image. Discrete Wavelet Transform (DWT) is applied to the host image to generate four subbands, and SVD is applied to each band to embed the watermark into the medical image. Here, SVM is used to classify between the ROI and RONI parts. Up to now, the data is embedded in the overall image, but a different scheme is presented by Manikandan et al., where the EPR data is embedded during encryption [22]. The original image is divided into n number of blocks. Then, for each block, the image is encrypted with hidden EPR data. Here, SVM is applied to classify between encrypted and normal blocks. Then the image is sent over the communication channel. This scheme also supports image recovery. Not only is authentication important, but also the detection of tampered areas plays a major role in medical imaging for further diagnosis [23, 24]. In the first step, a Wiener filter is applied to the host image to remove noise. After noise subtraction from the image, the noise pattern is estimated. The noise pattern is considered to classify the forged image. Then SVM and ELM are applied, and based on the score, the image is classified as forged or not. To classify images as forged or not, Zhang et al. also proposed a Krawtchouk moment [25]. This Krawtchouk helps distinguish between modified and normal images. Machine learning-based watermarking yields robustness against image processing attacks [26]. First, the medical image is classified into ROI and RONI using a Support Vector Machine (SVM) classifier. Then the watermark image is divided into two watermarks. Next, DWT is applied to the RONI part and converted into singular values using SVD. Finally, an XOR operation is performed for the watermark and embedded into the original image. This scheme is compared with two other methods to evaluate the performance of the proposed algorithm in terms of imperceptibility.

An invisible watermarking scheme is presented by Islam using SVM and LWT techniques [27]. Here, the original image is decomposed into 3 levels to obtain 3-level LWT subbands. Then, the selection of subbands is done. For the selected subband, randomization of coefficients is generated using Key 1. Then, it is divided into 2×2 blocks using Key 2. The difference is taken between two coefficients. On the other side, the reference watermark and signature are concatenated to form a binary watermark. Then, the coefficients are updated for each block. Finally, LWT is applied to obtain the watermarked image. A new transform is applied to embed the watermark to provide authentication for medical images [28]. Here, a hybrid technique is introduced using Tchebichef transform. To enhance the security, CAT mapping is used to scramble the watermark. Firstly, the original image is decomposed into two components that are sparse and low-rank using robust principal component analysis. Finally, DTT is used to embed the watermark. This scheme is imperceptible against various geometric attacks. Balamurugan also presents a hybrid watermark using SVM [29], where the original image is divided into ROI and RONI. The encrypted message is embedded into the ROI part. The encrypted message contains biometric keys generated by the iris. Transform domain methods are used to embed the encrypted message, and finally, a watermarked image is generated. Nowadays, collecting a medical-related dataset is very crucial due to its confidentiality. Kaissis proposed a secure and privacy-preserving algorithm using artificial intelligence for healthcare applications [30]. This scheme is resistant to various potential attacks. Securing medical images from attacks is still a challenge. Balasamy presented a pre-processing step [31]. In this step, noise is removed from the medical image and the median value is added for the noisy pixels. Then features are extracted to find the ROI part. To increase security, DWT is applied to the watermark, then SVD is applied to calculate the key component. This key component is embedded using DWT into the ROI. Clustering is also important in the case of medical imaging. Ouahi proposed KNN clustering to extract features from the image. The image is divided into 8×8 blocks, then DCT is applied to extract features from the original image. Further KNN clustering is used to select the features to embed. Next, the watermarked image is generated using the IDCT technique [32].

9.1.2 DEEP LEARNING

Kishore et al. present an idea about securing medical images using artificial neural networks (ANN) [33]. Here, the main idea is to alter the pixels of the image with a watermark. The altered pixels reduce the clarity of the image. ANN is used to reconstruct the pixels during transmission and watermarking of the image. The main goal of Kalaivani is to develop an effective watermarking method using a neural network to enhance data security [34]. This method utilizes the human visual system (HVS) to improve the invisibility of the watermarked data. The medical image is divided into a number of blocks, and for each block, a multiwavelet transform is applied. Subsequently, the neural network is used to create a more secure watermarked image using the Levenberg-Marquardt algorithm. However, there are trade-offs between visibility and robustness. Currently, there is no ideal solution or method for invisible watermarking [35]. In this study, Wong et al. proposed watermarking methods based on hybrid and deep learning techniques. The hybrid watermark includes DCT, DWT, and SVD. The watermark encoding is performed in string format into the original image. The encoded image is then subjected to 18 different attack methods, and transmission is carried out at this stage. Finally, the watermarked image is decoded, and the PSNR and NC values are calculated to visualize the results. To ensure that the watermarking process is reliable and undetectable, an iterative approach is proposed by Madhu [35]. Stationary wavelet transformation (SWT) and SVD are applied on both the host image and watermark image. Then embed the watermark into the original image. The watermarked image is then given as input to the CNN. This CNN distinguishes between the watermark image and tampered image. To enhance the security of medical images, VGG19, a deep learning model used by Han et al. [37], is employed. Features are extracted from the original image using VGG19. Fourier transform is applied to these features to build a feature matrix. To obtain a hash value, this feature matrix is input to the mean perceptual hashing algorithm. Then, the hash value is embedded into the original image and the watermarked image is scrambled using the perceptual hash value. Finally, the Hermite chaotic neural network is used to provide double protection. This algorithm ensures security against geometric attacks.

Not only authentication plays a role in medical imaging, identifying whether the suspected image is correct or not is also equally important. To differentiate between tampered and non-tampered images, Chen et al. proposed a lossless watermarking system [38]. The original watermark undergoes distortion processing, which distorts the watermarks. The distorted watermarks are then collected, labeled, and stored in a distorted dataset. This dataset is used for training to extract the watermark from the suspected medical image. Then WMnet is applied to the image to differentiate between tampered and non-tampered images. To provide authentication and protection for medical data, a novel fragile watermarking approach is proposed by Ali [39]. The original image is segmented into 3×3 blocks to generate a non-uniform code. LBP is applied to insert the watermark into the host image. The watermark includes the patient ID as a secret key. This algorithm is analyzed with two different datasets and is resilient to attacks. However, adversarial attacks remain an important problem to solve in medical image analysis. To address this issue, deep learning approaches are introduced by Apostolidis to protect medical images [40]. In this approach, Krawtchouk moments are calculated for the original image, generating a key set K1. Dither modulation is used to combine one signal with another to produce a set of generated key values, resulting in another key value K2. An XOR operation is performed between K1 and K2 to construct the watermark. Finally, the watermarked image is generated.

9.2 CONCLUSION

In recent years, artificial intelligence methods have been deployed in every dimension of human life. This includes machine learning (ML) and deep learning (DL) techniques that are quite adaptable to real-world situations, and the frameworks benefit from the learning process. ML and DL in medical imaging have significant implications for patient treatment. The fundamentals of ML and DL algorithms utilized in the field of healthcare are covered in this chapter. This chapter describes how to use these algorithms to address categorization and security-related problems associated with medical data. The categorization and security of diagnostic pictures are frequently handled by machine learning methods like SVM and NN. Many telemedicine applications use deep learning techniques, in particular CNN, to secure diagnostic pictures. According to this survey, we have found that many methods are created for specific uses, while others are still developing and have a lot of potential. It is essential to develop reliable and secure authentication techniques to safeguard the integrity and confidentiality of patients' sensitive medical data against unauthorized access and tampering.

KEYWORDS

- **authentication**
- **confidentiality**
- **deep learning**
- **integrity**
- **localization**
- **machine learning**
- **recovery**
- **tampering**

REFERENCES

1. Jannin, P., Grova, C., & Maurer, C. R. (2006). Model for defining and reporting reference-based validation protocols in medical image processing. *International Journal of Computer Assisted Radiology and Surgery*, *1*(2), 63–73. https://doi.org/10.1007/s11548-006-0042-y.
2. Michalski, R. S., Carbonell, J. G., & Mitchell, T. M. (Eds.). (2013). *Machine Learning: An Artificial Intelligence Approach*, 1–35. Springer Science & Business Media.

3. Norris, D. J. (2017). Machine learning: Deep learning. In *Beginning artificial intelligence with the Raspberry Pi* (pp. 211–247). Springer. https://doi.org/10.1007/978-1-4842-2980-6_8.
4. Jankowski, N., & Grochowski, M. (2004). Comparison of instances selection algorithms I. Algorithms survey. In *International Conference on Artificial Intelligence and Soft Computing* (pp. 598–603). Springer, Berlin, Heidelberg. https://doi.org/10.1007/978-3-540-24844-6_91.
5. Suzuki, K. (2012). Pixel-based machine learning in medical imaging. *Journal of Biomedical Imaging*, *2012*, 1. https://doi.org/10.1155/2012/427107.
6. Agarwal, T. K., Tiwari, M., & Lamba, S. S. (2014). Modified histogram-based contrast enhancement using homomorphic filtering for medical images. In *Advance Computing Conference (IACC), 2014 IEEE International* (pp. 819–823). IEEE. https://doi.org/10.1109/IAdCC.2014.6779394.
7. Fu, G., & Peng, H. (2007, September). Subsampling-based wavelet watermarking algorithm using support vector regression. In *EUROCON 2007-The International Conference on" Computer as a Tool"* (pp. 138–141). IEEE. https://doi.org/10.1109/EURCON.2007.4400587.
8. Peng, H., Wang, J., & Wang, W. (2010). Image watermarking method in multiwavelet domain based on support vector machines. *Journal of Systems and Software*, *83*(8), 1470–1477. https://doi.org/10.1016/j.jss.2010.01.041.
9. Sun, X., & Bo, S. (2010, June). A blind digital watermarking for color medical images based on PCA. In *2010 IEEE International Conference on Wireless Communications, Networking and Information Security* (pp. 421–427). IEEE. https://doi.org/10.1109/WCINS.2010.5541906.
10. Ramly, S., Aljunid, S. A., & Shaker Hussain, H. (2011, July). SVM-SS watermarking model for medical images. In *International Conference on Digital Enterprise and Information Systems* (pp. 372–386). Springer, Berlin, Heidelberg. https://doi.org/10.1007/978-3-642-22726-4_31.
11. Rathi, S. C., & Inamdar, V. S. (2012, May). Analysis of watermarking techniques for medical images preserving ROI. In *Computer Science & Information Technology (CS & IT 05) – open access – Computer Science Conference Proceedings (CSCP)* (pp. 297–308).
12. Alamgir, N., & Kim, J. M. (2013). Fuzzy clustering based medical image watermarking. *KIPS Transactions on Software and Data Engineering*, *2*(7), 487–494. https://doi.org/10.3745/KTSDE.2013.2.7.487.
13. Emami, M. S., & Omar, K. (2013). A low-cost method for reliable ownership identification of medical images using SVM and Lagrange duality. *Expert Systems with Applications*, *40*(18), 7579–7587. https://doi.org/10.1016/j.eswa.2013.07.034.
14. Mangaiyarkarasi, P., & Arulselvi, S. (2013). Medical image watermarking based on DWT and ICA for copyright protection. In *Recent Advancements in System Modelling Applications* (pp. 21–33). Springer, India. https://doi.org/10.1007/978-81-322-1495-7_2.
15. Joseph, A., & Deepa, S. S. (2015, November). An efficient watermarking-based integrity control system for medical images. In *2015 International Conference on Control Communication & Computing India (ICCC)* (pp. 357–361). IEEE. https://doi.org/10.1109/ICCC.2015.7432944.

16. Nguyen, T. H., & Duong, D. M. (2015, October). Reversible medical image watermarking technique based on choosing threshold values in histogram shifting. In *2015 Seventh International Conference on Knowledge and Systems Engineering (KSE)* (pp. 204–209). IEEE. https://doi.org/10.1109/KSE.2015.58.
17. Badshah, G., Liew, S. C., Zain, J. M., & Ali, M. (2016). Watermark compression in medical image watermarking using Lempel-Ziv-Welch (LZW) lossless compression technique. *Journal of Digital Imaging, 29*(2), 216–225. https://doi.org/10.1007/s10278-015-9850-3.
18. Singh, A., Raghuvanshi, N., Dutta, M. K., Burget, R., & Masek, J. (2016, June). An SVD based zero watermarking scheme for authentication of medical images for tele-medicine applications. In *2016 39th International Conference on Telecommunications and Signal Processing (TSP)* (pp. 511–514). IEEE. https://doi.org/10.1109/TSP.2016.7760918.
19. Suganya, R., & Kanagavalli, R. (2016). Tamper detection using watermarking scheme and K-mean clustering for bio-medical images. *International Journal for Modern Trends in Science and Technology, 2*, 180–185.
20. Dhavale, S. V. (2017). Robust embedding of patient ID in medical images for telemedicine applications. *Asian Journal for Convergence in Technology (AJCT), 3*, 2350–1146.
21. Rai, A., & Singh, H. V. (2017). SVM based robust watermarking for enhanced medical image security. *Multimedia Tools and Applications, 76*(18), 18605–18618. https://doi.org/10.1007/s11042-016-3819-7.
22. Manikandan, V. M., & Masilamani, V. (2018). Reversible data hiding scheme during encryption using machine learning. *Procedia Computer Science, 133*, 348–356. https://doi.org/10.1016/j.procs.2018.07.287.
23. Ghoneim, A., Muhammad, G., Amin, S. U., & Gupta, B. (2018). Medical image forgery detection for smart healthcare. *IEEE Communications Magazine, 56*(4), 33–37. https://doi.org/10.1109/MCOM.2018.1601307.
24. Solaiyappan, S., & Wen, Y. (2022). Machine learning based medical image deepfake detection: A comparative study. *Machine Learning with Applications, 8*, 100298. https://doi.org/10.1016/j.mlwa.2022.100298.
25. Zhang, X., Liu, X., Chen, Y., & Shu, H. (2018). Medical image blind integrity verification with krawtchouk moments. *International Journal of Biomedical Imaging, 2018*. https://doi.org/10.1155/2018/3068213.
26. Rai, A., & Singh, H. V. (2018). Machine learning-based robust watermarking technique for medical image transmitted over LTE network. *Journal of Intelligent Systems, 27*(1), 105–114. https://doi.org/10.1515/jisys-2017-0137.
27. Islam, M., Roy, A., & Laskar, R. H. (2020). SVM-based robust image watermarking technique in LWT domain using different sub-bands. *Neural Computing and Applications, 32*(5), 1379–1403. https://doi.org/10.1007/s00521-018-3763-7.
28. Noor, R., Khan, A., Sarfaraz, A., Mehmood, Z., & Cheema, A. M. (2019). Highly robust hybrid image watermarking approach using Tchebichef transform with secured PCA and CAT encryption. *Soft Computing, 23*(20), 9821–9829. https://doi.org/10.1007/s00500-018-3168-2.
29. Balamurugan, G., & Jayabharathy, J. (2020). A Hybrid Based Robust Watermarking Technique Using SVM. *AIJR Abstracts, 24*, 1–24.

30. Kaissis, G. A., Makowski, M. R., Rückert, D., & Braren, R. F. (2020). Secure, privacy-preserving and federated machine learning in medical imaging. *Nature Machine Intelligence, 2*(6), 305–311. https://doi.org/10.1038/s42256-020-00239-7.
31. Balasamy, K., & Shamia, D. (2021). Feature extraction-based medical image watermarking using fuzzy-based median filter. *IETE Journal of Research, 69,* 1–9. https://doi.org/10.1080/03772063.2021.1973496.
32. Ouahi, H., & Mazoul, A. (2021). Adaptive Image Watermarking based on K-NN Clustering. *American Academic Scientific Research Journal for Engineering, Technology, and Sciences, 76*(1), 253–263.
33. Kishore, P. V. V., Prajwal, K. S., Mohan, M. K., & Koteswarao, S. (2015, July). Medical image watermarking with ANN in wavelet domain. In *2015 IEEE International Conference on Electronics, Computing and Communication Technologies (CONECCT)* (pp. 1–6). IEEE. https://doi.org/10.1109/CONECCT.2015.7383841.
34. Kalaivani, K. (2017). An efficient watermarking scheme for medical data security with the aid of neural network. *Brazilian Archives of Biology and Technology, 59,* 1–12. https://doi.org/10.1590/1678-4324-2017160790.
35. Wong, Y. L., Loh, J. C., Li, C. Z., & Tan, C. W. (2021). A comparative study on medical image watermarking using hybrid approach and RIVAGAN. In *International Conference on Digital Transformation and Applications (ICDXA)* (Vol. 25, p. 26).
36. Madhu, B., & Holi, G. (2021). CNN approach for medical image authentication. *Indian Journal of Science and Technology, 14*(4), 351–360. https://doi.org/10.17485/ijst%2F2021%2Fv14i4%2F163114.
37. Han, B., Du, J., Jia, Y., & Zhu, H. (2021). Zero-Watermarking Algorithm for Medical Image Based on VGG19 Deep Convolution Neural Network. *Journal of Healthcare Engineering, 2021*, 1–12.
38. Chen, Y. P., Fan, T. Y., & Chao, H. C. (2021). Wmnet: a lossless watermarking technique using deep learning for medical image authentication. *Electronics, 10*(8), 932. https://doi.org/10.3390/electronics10080932.
39. Ali, Z., & Hussain, M. (2022). A Novel Fragile Zero-Watermarking Algorithm for Digital Medical Images. *Electronics, 11*(5), 710. https://doi.org/10.3390/electronics11050710.
40. Apostolidis, K. D., & Papakostas, G. A. (2022). Digital Watermarking as an Adversarial Attack on Medical Image Analysis with Deep Learning. *Journal of Imaging, 8*(6), 155. https://doi.org/10.3390/jimaging8060155.

CHAPTER 10

Data-Driven Analytics for Healthcare: Artificial Intelligence and Machine Learning for Medical Diagnostics

B. MALAVIKA,[1] A. V. SENTHIL KUMAR,[1] G. VANISHREE,[2] and MEENAKSHI SHARMA[3]

[1]*Department of MCA, Hindusthan College of Arts and Science, Coimbatore, Tamil Nadu, India*

[2]*Faculty, IBS, Bangalore, Karnataka, India*

[3]*Assistant Professor-SS, University of Petroleum and Energy Studies, Dehradun, Uttarakhand, India*

ABSTRACT

The idea of Learning Health Systems is the acquisition of energy as an increasing number of digital healthcare statistics will become an increasing number of available data. The core concept is to allow getting to know from the collective experience of a healthcare transport network as recorded within the observational statistics, to iteratively enhance the quality of healthcare as the healthcare is being supplied in an actual global setting. In association with this revelation, a whole lot of current research effort has been dedicated to exploring system learning, data visualization, and data mining methodologies that can be used to originate actual global proof from diverse resources of healthcare statistics to provide personalized choice support for healthcare transport and healthcare management systems.

Data-Driven Analytics for Healthcare: Artificial Intelligence and Machine Learning for Medical Diagnostics. Meghna Sharma, Priyanka Vashisht, A. V. Senthil Kumar, Chitra Singh, and Abdelmalek Amine (Eds.)

The major purpose of this research is to study data-driven analytics applied in the field of medical diagnostics and how artificial intelligence and machine learning algorithms are implemented in the healthcare industry. Tableau is the data visualization tool used, and the algorithm is the simple exponential algorithm. This simple exponential algorithm is used to find the forecast results with respect to time. Thus, the results of this study reveal the prediction of negative test case count. For plotting purposes, bar graphs and line plots are used.

10.1 INTRODUCTION

In contemporary days, artificial intelligence has swiftly developed in standards of automated methodologies, hardware applications, and techniques in several regions. This study precises the maximum current enhancements in artificial intelligence and machine learning, and the sensible techniques of artificial intelligence and machine learning in biomedicine such as disorder diagnosis, existence support, biomedical studies, and biomedical data processing. Once a set of rules learns the way to use data, it can carry out mechanically, which is the important key benefit of system learning. Cardiac diseases, neural problems, and most cancers are the predominant infection areas that take advantage of artificial intelligence and machine learning technology. The intention of this study is to keep track of recent research findings, discover technological availability, appraise the substantial potential of artificial intelligence and machine learning in biomedicine, and encourage biomedical investigators [28]. Like artificial intelligence and machine learning itself, it can be argued that its application to biomedicine remains in its infancy. Further development and discoveries push the bounds and within the foreseeable future, the potential of artificial intelligence and machine learning is expected to continue to increase [38].

10.1.1 DATA ANALYTICS

The data analytics can be defined as a study of analyzing the raw facts to conclude with the decisions. There are a number of methods and procedures of data analytics which have been automated to the algorithms and mechanical procedures which operate on the raw facts to support human needs. As a definition, “Data analytics is the science of analyzing raw data to make conclusions about that information.” Data analytics supports a business enterprise to promote optimized performance, with more efficiency, producing more profit, and to prepare strategic-oriented decisions. The processes and techniques of data analytics are always automated to ease the task of the human [1]. Figure 10.1 shows steps in data analysis.

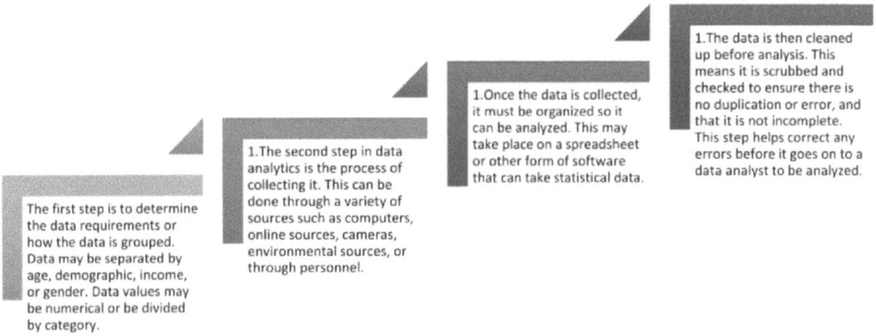

FIGURE 10.1 Steps in data analysis.

The first step is to decide the records necessities or how the records are clustered. Data can be separated by gender, income, demographic, or age. Data values can be numerical or divided by category [28]. The second step in records analytics is the method of gathering it. This can be done through a variety of sources including computers, online resources, cameras, environmental resources, or personnel. Once the records are collected, they should be prepared for analysis. This can be done on a spreadsheet or other software that can handle statistical records. The records are then cleaned up before analysis [29]. This means they are checked and scrubbed to ensure there are no errors or duplications, and that they are not incomplete [42]. This step helps correct any mistakes before the data is passed on to a data analyst for evaluation. Data analytics relies on various software tools such as data visualization tools, spreadsheets, and reporting tools like data mining programs, or open-source languages for extensive data manipulation. Data analytics is an extensive term that incorporates numerous varieties of data analysis. Any form of statistics may be subjected to data analytics strategies to gain insights that can be used to enhance things. Data analytics strategies can monitor trends and metrics that could otherwise be lost in the mass of data [27]. This data can later be used to optimize processes to increase the overall performance of a system or an enterprise. For example, production groups often record the work queue, runtime, and downtime for various machines, and then data analysts can analyze the information to improve the workloads, so the machines perform at their peak capacity. Data analytics can do much more than just point out holdups in production. Gaming companies use data analytics to set reward schedules for players that keep the majority of players active in the game. Content companies use some of the same data analytics to keep people engaged by reorganizing, clicking on, or watching content to get another view or another click [26].

10.2 DATA ANALYTICS FOR HEALTHCARE

The healthcare enterprise generates a great quantity of facts but struggles to transform that data into understandings that enhance patient outcomes and operational efficiencies. Data analytics in healthcare is meant to help providers overcome barriers to the effective application of data-derived intelligence; Making healthcare data easier to share among colleagues and external partners, and easier to visualize for public consumption, Providing accurate data-driven predictions in real time to enable healthcare providers to respond more quickly to changing healthcare markets and environments, and Enhancing data innovation and collaboration among healthcare teams to transform analytics-ready information into business-ready data by systematizing low-impact data management tasks [21]. The software tools used in analytics fall into three popular categories:

- Software that acquires the information from resources that encompass affected person case files, surveys, and device-to-device information transfers;
- Programs that validate, clean, and examine the information in reaction to a particular studies question; and
- Software that shapes at the outcomes of the evaluation to signify numerous movements to obtain unique healthcare goals.

Along with analyzing, collecting, and decoding information, analytics software program should steady the information and the evaluation outcomes whilst making sure that the healthcare specialists who'll benefit from the insights have equipped get access to the information in a shape that they are able to without difficulty use of their work (Figure 10.2).

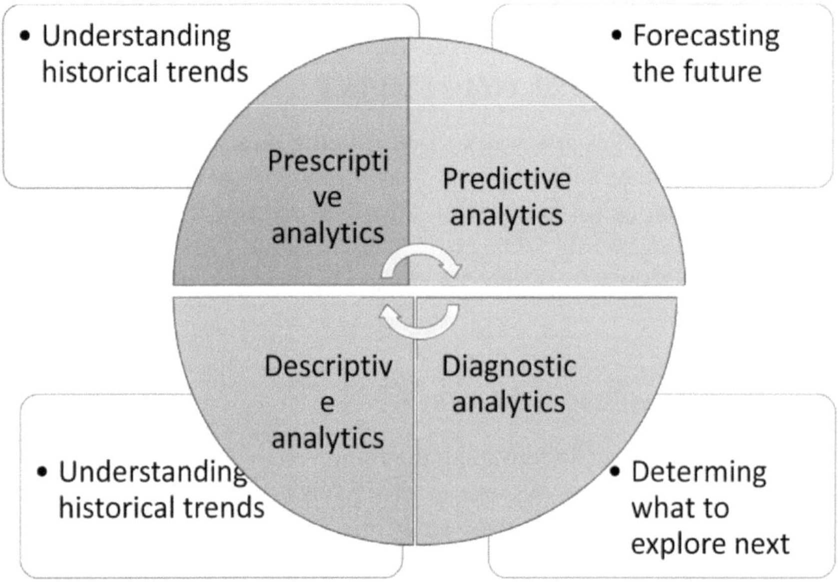

FIGURE 10.2 The four types of healthcare data analytics.

There are a number of approaches to data analytics such as prescriptive analytics, predictive analytics, diagnostic analytics, and descriptive analytics [27]. Predictive analysis describes "what is going to happen?" prescriptive analytics provides the solution for the question "what should be done next?" diagnostic analytics focuses on "why something happened?" and descriptive analytics gives a clear idea of "what happened?"

10.2.1 PREDICTIVE STATISTICS ANALYTICS

Predictive analytics is the most commonly used type of data analytics. Businesses use predictive analytics to identify trends, correlations, and causation. This group can be further broken down into statistical modeling and predictive modeling, but it's important to understand that the two go hand in hand. For example, an advertising campaign for t-shirts on Facebook could use predictive analytics to determine how closely conversion rate correlates with a target audience's geographical location, interests, and income bracket. Predictive modeling could then be used to analyze the data for one or more target audiences and provide potential sales values for each demographic [33].

10.2.2 PRESCRIPTIVE DATA ANALYTICS

Prescriptive analytics is where artificial intelligence and big data integrate to help predict outcomes and identify which actions to take. This category of analytics can be further broken down into random testing and optimization [31]. Leveraging advancements in machine learning, prescriptive analytics can help answer questions such as "What is the best course of action?"

10.2.3 DIAGNOSTIC DATA ANALYTICS

While not as exciting as predicting the future, analyzing data from the past can serve an important purpose in managing one's business. Diagnostic data analytics is the process of analyzing data to understand cause and effect or why an event occurred. Techniques such as data mining, data discovery, correlations, and drill down are commonly used. Diagnostic data analytics help answer questions about why something happened. Like the other categories, it is also broken down into more specific categories: results and indicators and query and drill downs [41]. Drill downs and queries are used to obtain more details from a report. For example, a sales representative who closed significantly fewer deals in one month. A drill down could reveal fewer workdays, due to a two-week vacation. Discoveries and alerts notify of a potential issue before it occurs, for instance, an alert about a decrease in staff hours, which could result in a decrease in closed deals. Diagnostic data analytics can also be used to "discover" information such as the most qualified candidate for a new role at a company [22].

10.2.4 DESCRIPTIVE STATISTICS ANALYTICS

Descriptive analytics are the backbone of reporting—it's not possible to have BI (business intelligence) equipment and dashboards without it. It addresses simple questions of "what, when, where, and how many."

Again, descriptive analytics may be further separated into categories: canned reports and ad hoc reporting. A canned report is one that has been designed previously and includes data about a given topic. An example of this is a monthly report sent by the ad agency or ad group that details performance metrics for your current advertising efforts [24].

10.3 ARTIFICIAL INTELLIGENCE AND ITS APPLICATIONS

Artificial intelligence can be defined as "the simulation of human intelligence processes by machines, especially computer systems. Specific applications of artificial intelligence include expert systems, natural language processing, speech recognition, and machine vision." As the hype around artificial intelligence has increased, companies have been scrambling to explain how their services and products use artificial intelligence. Often what they refer to as artificial intelligence is actually one aspect of artificial intelligence, such as machine learning. Artificial intelligence requires a foundation of specialized hardware and software for training and developing machine learning algorithms. "No one programming language is synonymous with artificial intelligence," but some, including Java, Python, and R, are common [32].

In general, artificial intelligence structures operations by consuming massive amounts of categorized training data, analyzing the data for correlations and patterns, and using those patterns to make predictions about future states. In this way, a chatbot that is fed examples of text chats can learn to produce realistic exchanges with people, or a photo recognition system can learn to identify and define objects in images by studying millions of examples [24]. Figure 10.3 shows some applications of AI in healthcare.

A brief description of all the applications is given as follows:

1. **Clinical Trials:** Artificial intelligence can discover appropriate candidates for clinical trials by analyzing medical data and social media content. Trial recruitment can be accelerated by using artificial intelligence technology to notify medical staff and patients about trial opportunities, as well as by shortening entry criteria to be more accessible for potential participants. While artificial intelligence has shown potential benefits, overall data management and reduction of bias in data are needed to effectively utilize artificial intelligence [35].

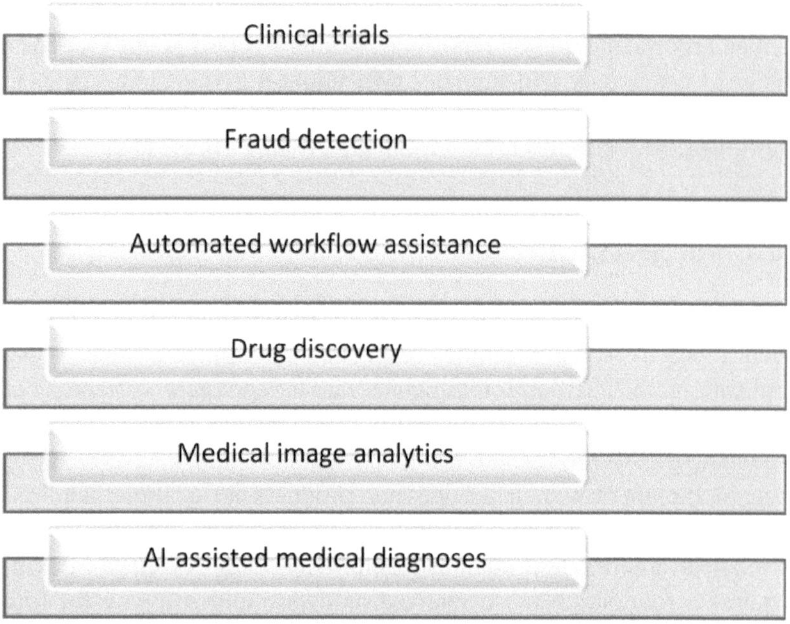

FIGURE 10.3 Applications of artificial intelligence in healthcare.

2. **Fraud Detection:** The healthcare sector generates vast amounts of data daily, from patient diagnoses to diagnostic imagery stored digitally on hospital servers. It's more data than a human statistician — or even a team of them — could hope to sift through. Artificial intelligence and machine learning systems can sort, categorize, and analyze large amounts of data in a fraction of the time. Artificial intelligence systems also tend to be more accurate because they eliminate the possibility of human error [35]. These systems are much more efficient than human analysts because the constraints of biology do not hold them back. When programmed correctly, they have nearly infinite memory and processing capacity, something not even the most brilliant human mind can match. Instead of looking at recent data, an artificial intelligence system can sift through years of patient records and related data in seconds, identifying similar patterns a human analyst might overlook [2].

3. **Automated Workflow Assistance:** Healthcare or medical workflow automation aims at enhancing the capability of the healthcare system with the goal of reshuffling the various processes involved

to provide the best experience possible for the patients. Workflow automation focuses on processes in both administrative and operational ways. The use of technology to automate medical workflows helps standardize high-volume workflows to improve efficiency in every way possible. By enhancing medical or healthcare workflow, healthcare sectors will be able to get things done in less time, collaborate, and communicate effectively to deliver better care for patients [36].

4. **Drug Discovery:** Artificial intelligence could assist medical sectors in bringing drugs to market faster. Artificial intelligence today not only aids in gene-sequencing efforts but is also being trained to predict drug effectiveness and side effects, and to manage the vast amounts of data and information that support almost all pharmaceutical innovation [15].

5. **Medical Image Analytics:** Artificial intelligence increasingly supports finding hidden insights into medical decision-making, connecting patients with sources for self-management, and extracting meaning from formerly unstructured, inaccessible records assets. Medical imaging records are one of the richest sources of information about patients and are often complex. With "megapixel upon megapixel" of data packed into the results from MRIs, CAT scans, X-rays, and other testing modalities, combing through extremely high-resolution images can be challenging even for the most skilled medical experts [30].

6. **AI-Assisted Medical Diagnosis:** The use of AI is rapidly growing in the medical field, particularly in diagnostics and treatment management. To date, there has been a wide range of research into how artificial intelligence can assist in medical decisions and improve physicians' judgment. Correct diagnosis is a crucial aspect of global healthcare systems. In the United States, about 5% of outpatients receive an incorrect diagnosis, with errors being particularly common for serious medical conditions, posing the risk of significant patient harm. In recent years, Artificial Intelligence and machine learning have emerged as powerful tools for aiding diagnosis. This technology could revolutionize healthcare by providing more accurate diagnoses. Scientists at Babylon, a

global tech company specializing in digital health, discovered a new way to use machine learning to diagnose diseases. They developed new Artificial Intelligence symptom checkers that they believe could help reduce diagnostic errors in primary care [37].

10.4 MACHINE LEARNING AND ITS APPLICATIONS

From playing a crucial function in patient care, billing, and clinical records, these days technology is permitting healthcare systems experts to expand change IP capitalization, staffing models, offer smart healthcare systems, and decreasing administrative and deliver costs. Machine learning in healthcare systems is one such location that is seeing slow recognition within the healthcare systems innovativeness [14]. Google recently developed a "machine-learning algorithm" to discover "cancerous tumors in mammograms," and scholars at Stanford University are using deep learning to discover skin cancer. ML is already providing assistance in numerous conditions in healthcare systems. Machine learning in healthcare systems allows to analyze hundreds of different records factors and suggest outcomes, provide timely risk scores, unique resource allocation, and has many other applications [11] (Figure 10.4).

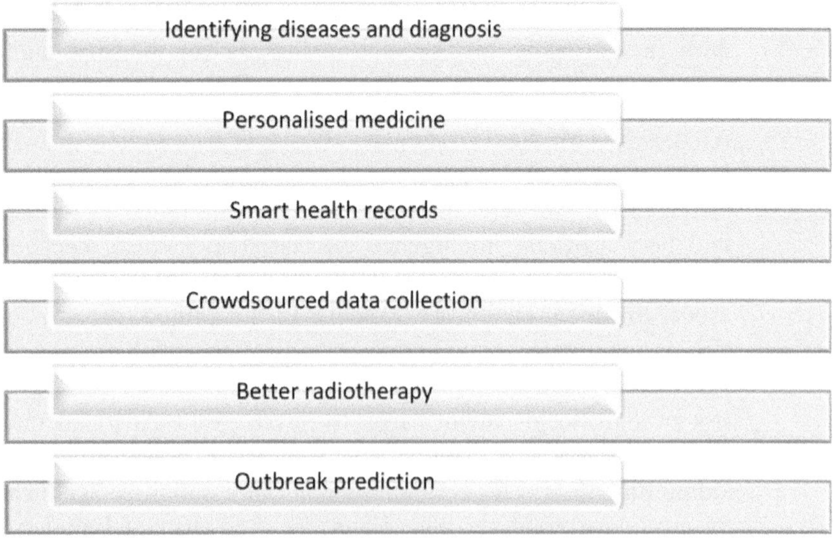

FIGURE 10.4 Applications of machine learning in healthcare.

An increasing number of developing variety of packages of device gaining knowledge of in healthcare permits the users to glimpse at a future wherein data, analysis, and innovation work together to assist infinite patients deprived of them ever understanding it. Soon, it'll be common to discover machine learning primarily based totally packages embedded with real-time patient data available from distinct healthcare systems in more than one country, thereby growing the efficacy of new treatment options which had been unavailable before [13]. Step by step explanation of each application is discussed in subsections.

10.4.1 IDENTIFYING DISEASES AND DIAGNOSIS

One of the most important Machine Learning applications in healthcare is the identification and analysis of diseases and conditions that may otherwise be considered hard to diagnose. This can include anything from cancers that are difficult to detect during the early stages, to other genetic diseases. IBM Watson Genomics is a prime example of how integrating cognitive computing with genome-based tumor sequencing can help in making a quick diagnosis. The biopharma giant is leveraging Artificial Intelligence to develop therapeutic treatments in areas such as oncology. "Predicting Response to Depression Treatment" aims to develop a commercially viable way to diagnose and provide treatment in typical medical conditions [9].

10.4.2 PERSONALIZED MEDICINE

Personalized treatments can not only be more effective by combining individual health with predictive analytics but are also ripe for further research and improved disease assessment. Currently, doctors are limited to choosing from a specific set of diagnoses or estimating the risk to the patient based on the symptomatic data and available genetic information. However, machine learning in medicine is making great strides, and IBM Watson Oncology is at the forefront of this movement by using patient medical records to help generate multiple treatment options [27].

10.4.3 SMART HEALTH RECORDS

Maintaining up-to-date fitness data is a comprehensive process, and while technology has played its part in simplifying the data access procedure, the fact is that even now, most of the processes take a lot of time to complete [20]. The main function of machine learning in healthcare is to streamline processes to save money, effort, and time. Document classification methods using support vector machines and machine learning-based OCR recognition techniques are slowly gaining traction, including MATLAB's and Google's Cloud Vision API machine learning-based handwriting recognition technology [4]. MIT is currently at the forefront of developing the next generation of intelligent health data, which will incorporate ML-based tools from the ground up to assist with diagnosis, medical treatment recommendations, etc.

10.4.4 CROWDSOURCED DATA COLLECTION

Crowdsourcing is all the rage within the clinical field nowadays, allowing researchers and practitioners to access a substantial amount of data uploaded by individuals based on their own consent [26]. This live health data has significant implications for how treatment could be perceived in the future. "Apple's Research Kit" enables users to access interactive applications that utilize Machine Learning-based facial recognition to attempt to address Parkinson's and Asperger's disease. IBM recently partnered with Decipher to Medtronic, accrue, and make available insulin and diabetes data in real-time based on the crowdsourced data. With the advancements being made on the Internet of Things, the healthcare industry continues to discover new ways to utilize this data and address difficult-to-diagnose cases, aiding in the overall advancement of medicine and diagnosis [19].

10.4.5 BETTER RADIOTHERAPY

One of the most desirable applications of machine learning in healthcare is in the field of Radiology. Medical image analysis has many different variables that can arise at any specific moment. There are many cancer foci, lesions, etc., which cannot be clearly demonstrated by the complex equations [22]. Since Machine Learning-based algorithms learn from the collection of various samples available on hand, it becomes easier to diagnose and identify the variables. One of the very popular advantages of ML in clinical image analysis is the classification of items such as lesions into categories such as abnormal or normal, non-lesion or lesion, etc. "Google's DeepMind Health" is actively assisting researchers at University College London Hospitals NHS Foundation Trust in developing algorithms that can detect the difference between healthy and cancerous tissue and improve radiation therapy for the same [39].

10.4.6 OUTBREAK PREDICTION

Machine Learning assists to collate these facts and expect everything from malaria outbreaks to extreme continual infectious illnesses. Forecasting these outbreaks is useful in third-world nations as they lack essential scientific infrastructure and academic systems [10]. A primary example of this is ProMED-mail, an Internet-based broadcasting platform that monitors developing illnesses and emerging ones and provides outbreak reports in real-time [18].

10.5 LITERATURE REVIEW

An investigation was conducted on automatic surveillance strategies for health-related contaminations. In that evaluation, researchers have defined how automated surveillance structures based on ML algorithms deliver more advantageous overall performance and dependability compared to manual surveillance approaches. Another finding of this evaluation is that the use of regression patterns can enhance the sensitivity and performance of surveillance plans [5]. There are a few challenges that need to be addressed in the near upcoming studies including case-blend adjustment, post-discharge surveillance, and quantification of tool operation. "BRONCHIOLITIS" is a lung infection that is commonly seen in young children and infants. Another researcher reviewed this disease along with RSV (respiratory syncytial virus), an infection that can be an origin cause of bronchiolitis. The systematic review provides some insights into predictive modeling and also mentioned how ML can be used to overcome barriers of predictive modeling. "SEPSIS" is a dangerous condition that occurs due to the body's response to infection, leading to inflammation that results in multiple organ failures simultaneously. A later conducted a systematic review to analyze the current trends in sepsis detection in hospitals [17].

Researchers have examined diverse sepsis detection marking structures and screening equipment together with their advantages and disadvantages in preferred medical institution wards. Finally, they located biomarkers and digital fitness information may have a big impact in predicting sepsis. They suggested a few disadvantages in recurring blood way of life checking out for sepsis detection. To analyze appropriate automated sepsis detection techniques, they examined seven molecular technologies that make use of blood samples. In that observation, they have mentioned the numerous future and present trends. Additionally, they have analyzed the effect of ML algorithms with digital clinical information in sepsis detection. They conclude that by merging diverse technologies, the detection method can be enhanced and the risk of using the incorrect antibiotic can be reduced [6].

Initially, the research used conventional feature extraction strategies for analysis. Amongst those strategies, the best ones are normally dependent on the fusion of more than one biological function and multi-model imaging data. Later, they used a mixed kernel method to fuse cerebral spinal fluids (CSFs), positron emission tomography (PET), and structural magnetic resonance imaging MRI functions and carried out an SVM (support vector machine) classifier to perform binary classification. Another researcher named Tong carried out a graph combination technique and organized a unified graph for classification by combining the best similarity vectors. These vectors were obtained by calculating pairwise similarities of functions [43].

10.6 METHODOLOGY

Research methodology refers to the real-world "how" of any specified section of studies. Specifically, it's about how a researcher analytically innovates an observation to ensure legitimate and dependable outcomes that address the study's objectives and aims [29]. For example, how did the researcher go about deciding:

- What information to acquire (and what data to ignore)?
- Where to acquire it from (in studies, that is called "sampling design")?
- How to acquire it (that is called "data collection methods")?
- How to examine it (that is called "data analysis methods")?

In this study, the author has used a tool called Tableau, which is known as one of the most recommended data visualization tools frequently used for business intelligence and data analysis. Tableau is considered superior when compared with Excel sheets because Tableau provides powerful dashboards and interactive visuals [8]. Figure 10.5 illustrates a screenshot from the data loading page of Tableau. There are many advantages to using Tableau, such as data visualization, scheduling or notification of reports, Tableau's ability to handle large amounts of data, Tableau Company Strategy, responsive dashboards, and quickly create interactive visualizations [40].

10.6.1 ALGORITHM USED

The algorithm is defined as "a procedure used for solving a problem or performing a computation." The algorithm used in this study is Exponential Smoothing. Exponential smoothing is a "time series forecasting technique" for univariate records that may be prolonged to guide records with a systematic pattern or seasonal component. It is an effective forecasting technique that can be used as an alternative to the popular "Box-Jenkins ARIMA" family of methods [7] (Figure 10.6).

- **Algorithm:**
  - **Step 1:** Data collection.
  - **Step 2:** Pre-processing data.
  - **Step 3:** Create class.
  - **Step 4:** Fit model.
  - **Step 5:** Make prediction.

Single Exponential Smoothing, SES for short, also known as Simple Exponential Smoothing, is a time series forecasting technique for univariate records without a pattern or seasonality. It requires a single parameter, known as alpha (α), also referred to as the smoothing coefficient or smoothing factor. This parameter controls the rate at which the influence of the observations at previous time steps decreases exponentially. Alpha is often set to a value between 1 and 0. Larger values imply that the model will focus more on the most recent past observations, while smaller values mean that more of the data is considered when making a prediction [16]. Eqn. (1) provides the formula for exponential smoothing.

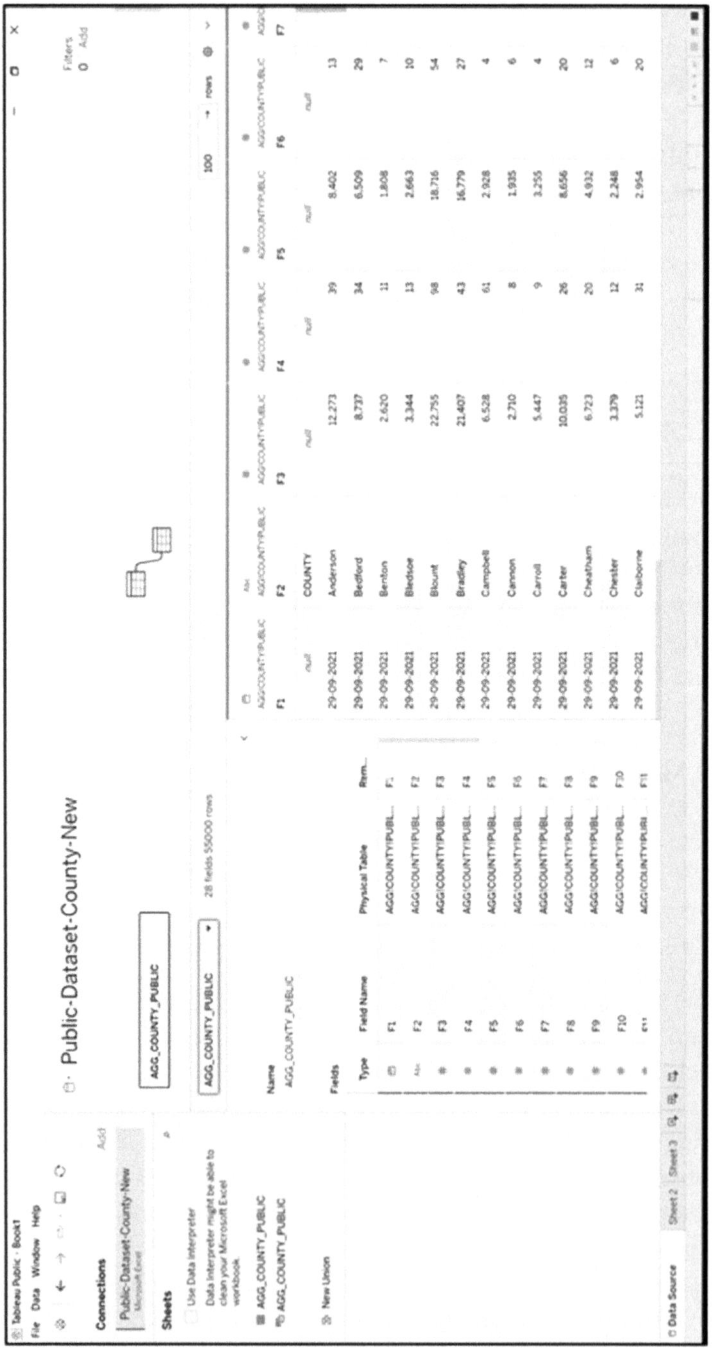

FIGURE 10.5 Tableau tool loading a dataset.

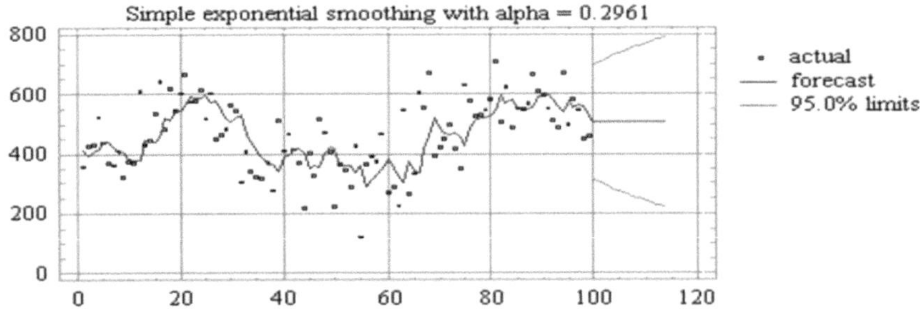

FIGURE 10.6 Single exponential soothing.

Formula:

$$S_t = \alpha y_{t-1} + (1-\alpha) S_{t-1} \quad (1)$$

Where;S_t stands for exponential smoothing; $\propto$ stands for the smoothing constant; t stands for the time period; and y denotes a constant which is selected with respect to $\propto$.

10.6.2 DATA DESCRIPTION

The above dataset shown in Figure 10.7 is a file which is in the format of CSV (comma-separated values) file. This dataset contains different countries of US which have their own test counts such as total cases reported, positive count, negative counts, new tests, deaths, active cases, recovered, and so on (Table 10.1).

TABLE 10.1 Dataset (Public-Dataset-Country-Name)

DATE – Dataset of countries on that particular date
COUNTRY – County of residence of the patient
TOTALCASES – Total number of confirmed and probable cases reported to TDH for the specific age range/age group category (TOTALCONFIRMED +TOTAL_PROBABLE)
NEW_CASES – Difference in a number of cases since previous day
TOTAL_CONFIRMED – Total number of confirmed COVID-19 cases, defined as having positive polymerase chain reaction (PCR) diagnostic tests reported to TDH
NEW_CONFIRMED – Difference in number of positive tests reported to TDH since previous day

TABLE 10.1 *(Continued)*

TOTAL_PROBABLE – Total Number of probable COVID Cases
NEW_PROBABLE – Difference in number of probable cases since previous day
POS_TESTS – Total number of positive polymerase chain reaction (PCR) diagnostic tests reported to TDH
NEWPOSTESTS – New number of positive polymerase chain reaction (PCR) diagnostic tests reported to TDH since the previous day
NEG_TESTS – Total number of negative polymerase chain reaction (PCR) diagnostic tests reported to TDH
NEW_NEG_TESTS – New number of negative polymerase chain reaction (PCR) diagnostic tests reported to TDH since the previous day
TOTAL_TESTS – Total number of positive and negative PCR tests reported to TDH (POSTESTS + NEGTESTS)
NEW_TESTS – Difference in number of tests reported to TDH since previous day
NEW_DEATHS – Difference in the number of deaths since previous day based on the date of public reporting (yesterday))
TOTAL_DEATHS – Total number of COVID-related deaths (TOTALCONFIRMED + TOTALPROBABLE) reported to TDH to date
NEW_ACTIVE (TOTAL Active (today) – TOTAL Active (yesterday))
TOTAL_ACTIVE (TOTALCASES – (TOTALDEATHS + TOTALINACTIVERECOVERED)) – Active cases are COVID-19 (TOTAL_ CONFIRMED + TOTAL_PROBABLE) cases who are not classified as inactive/ recovered and are not deceased
NEW_INACTIVE_RECOVERED (TOTALINACTIVERECOVERED (today) – TOTALINACTIVERECOVERED (yesterday))
TOTAL_INACTIVE_RECOVERED – Total Number of inactive/recovered COVID cases
NEW_HOSPITALIZED-TOTALHosp (today) – TOTALHosp (yesterday)
TOTAL_HOSPITALIZED – Total number of COVID cases (TOTALCONFIRMED + TOTALPROBABLE) who report ever being hospitalized for their illness
TOTAL_DEATHS_BY_DOD – Total number of deaths to date with known day of death

10.7 RESULTS AND DISCUSSIONS

The most important section of a research-oriented study is the results and discussions. It contains all the plots obtained during the study. This section helps the researcher to conclude and also provides an idea for the next researchers. In this study, the results are obtained using the tool called "Tableau" (Figure 10.8).

COUNTY	TOTAL_CASES	NEW_CASES	TOTAL_CONFIRMED	NEW_CONFIRMED	TOTAL_PROBABLE	NEW_PROBABLE	POS_TESTS	NEW_POS_TESTS	NEG_TESTS	NEW_NEG_TESTS	TOTAL_TESTS	NEW_TESTS	NEW_DEATHS	TOTAL_DEATHS	NEW_ACTIVE	TOTAL_ACTIVE	NEW_INACTIVE_RECOVERED	TOTAL_INACTIVE_RECOVERED	NEW_HOSPITALIZED	TOTAL_HOSPITALIZED	TOTAL_DEATHS_BY_DOD
Anderson	12273	39	8402	13	3871	26	9392	14	77828	191	87220	205	2	199	-29	519	66	11555	0	259	199
Bedford	8737	34	6509	29	2228	5	7458	31	40476	110	47934	141	0	148	3	274	31	8315	0	226	148
Benton	2620	11	1808	7	812	4	1984	10	11928	65	13912	75	0	44	-5	148	16	2428	0	77	44
Bledsoe	3344	13	2663	10	681	3	2839	10	19946	42	22785	52	0	13	3	101	10	3230	0	56	13
Blount	22755	98	18716	54	4039	44	20467	58	100896	293	121363	351	2	243	-21	991	117	21521	0	610	243
Bradley	21407	43	16779	27	4628	16	19032	35	89993	158	109025	193	1	172	-39	685	81	20550	0	813	172
Campbell	6528	61	2928	4	3600	57	3247	5	28859	58	32106	63	0	71	22	565	39	5892	0	135	71
Cannon	2710	8	1935	6	775	2	2139	7	11913	25	14052	32	0	38	-2	92	10	2580	0	77	38
Carroll	5447	9	3255	4	2192	5	3747	4	24531	45	28278	49	0	95	-15	265	24	5087	0	157	95
Carter	10035	26	8656	20	1379	6	9478	24	52457	135	61935	159	0	203	-39	417	65	9415	0	392	203
Cheatham	6723	20	4932	12	1791	8	5549	18	36647	106	42196	124	0	64	-7	269	27	6390	0	163	64
Chester	3379	12	2248	6	1131	6	2597	7	16455	27	19052	34	0	66	4	129	8	3184	0	66	66
Claiborne	5121	31	2954	20	2167	11	3196	23	28861	58	32057	81	0	90	-2	337	33	4694	0	112	90
Clay	1438	4	973	3	465	1	1106	3	6622	19	7728	22	0	35	-7	70	11	1333	0	54	35
Cocke	6944	39	4088	16	2856	23	4543	18	28461	76	33004	94	0	104	1	321	38	6519	0	133	104
Coffee	10107	60	6515	25	3592	35	7767	35	56772	155	64539	190	0	144	6	407	54	9556	0	247	144
Crockett	3262	6	1788	2	1474	4	2020	2	10061	15	12081	17	0	59	-4	79	10	3124	0	42	59
Cumberland	10549	55	8255	42	2294	13	9344	49	59426	170	68770	219	1	200	-1	427	55	9922	0	275	200
Davidson	116922	326	107613	299	9309	27	130260	348	1263915	3281	1394175	3629	2	1095	-54	3565	378	112262	2	2912	1095
Decatur	2336	4	1521	2	815	2	1765	4	12715	13	14480	17	0	42	-7	91	11	2203	0	62	42
Dekalb	4051	12	2864	8	1187	4	3260	9	21006	55	24266	64	1	64	-4	133	15	3854	0	104	64
Dickson	9958	35	7193	18	2765	17	8318	21	47163	138	55481	159	1	159	-3	320	37	9479	0	281	159
Dyer	7926	26	4559	7	3367	19	5101	7	26694	35	31795	42	0	134	-7	250	33	7542	0	160	134
Fayette	7055	16	5656	10	1399	6	6929	10	48725	112	55654	122	0	97	-9	186	25	6772	0	266	97
Fentress	3432	23	2697	14	735	9	3054	19	16970	31	20024	50	0	59	10	165	13	3208	0	132	59

FIGURE 10.7 Sample dataset.

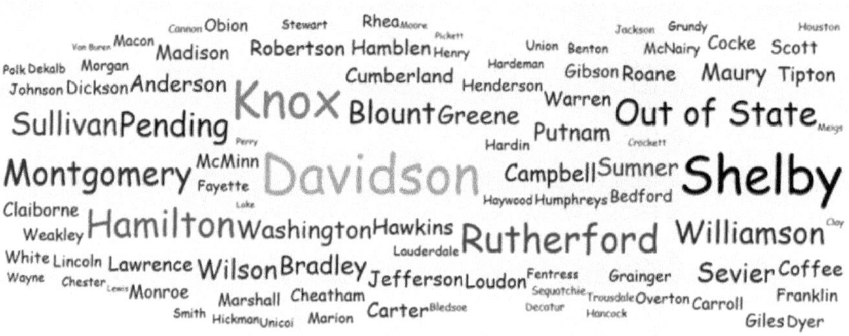

FIGURE 10.8 Word cloud of the COVID cases in the countries in US.

Figure 10.8 illustrates the word cloud of the COVID-19 cases reported in the countries of the US. With analysis, the researcher found that Shelby has many death cases comparatively. The dark red denotes the largest death cases, yellow denotes average death cases, and blue has the least number of death cases due to COVID-19 [25].

In the bar graph as shown in Figure 10.9, the darker shade (green) signifies a large count of deaths, which is seen in the mid area (November to January). The lighter shade represents lower death rates. The gradual growth is in the count of positive cases, but it decreased in the month of October 2021. With this data, the forecast is plotted in Figures 10.10 and 10.11 [34].

Figure 10.10 gives the prediction of death rates week by week. The first section, labeled "Actual," contains the data available in the dataset up to the month of July 2021. The section below, labeled "Estimate," shows a forecast plot of the death rates. Based on the plot, the author concludes that the death rates are decreasing over time [3].

Figure 10.11 has a forecast of negative tests. Until September 2021, it has an alternate line plot which shows a possibility of more positive cases. However, in the "estimate" section, the number of negative tests is increasing, indicating that the number of COVID positive patients will decrease, leading to a fall in the death rate as well [23].

10.8 CONCLUSION

The contemporary observation offers a quick description of how machine learning can assist in classifying, segmenting, and detecting distinct

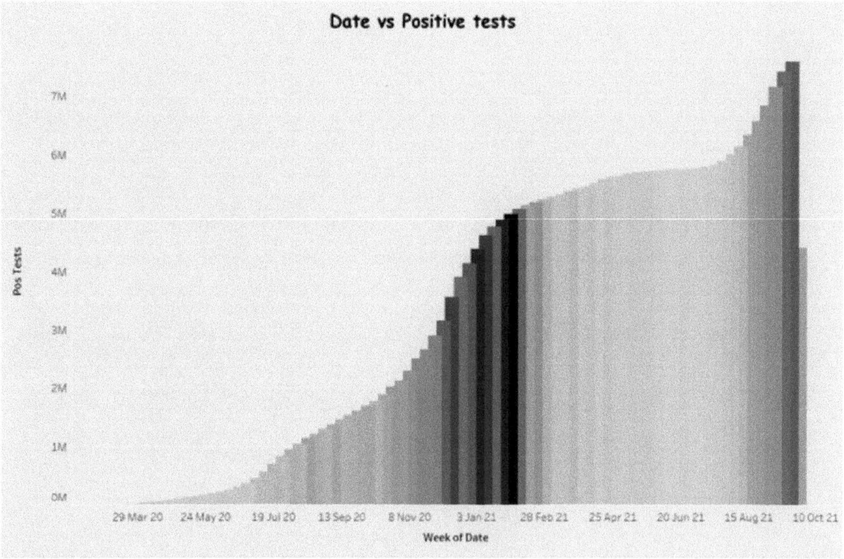

FIGURE 10.9 Bar graph of the date and positive tests.

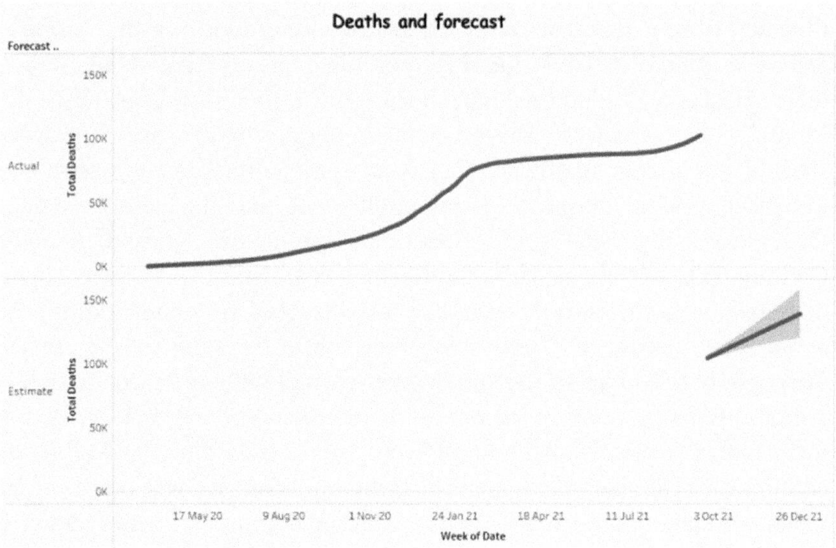

FIGURE 10.10 Forecast of death rates.

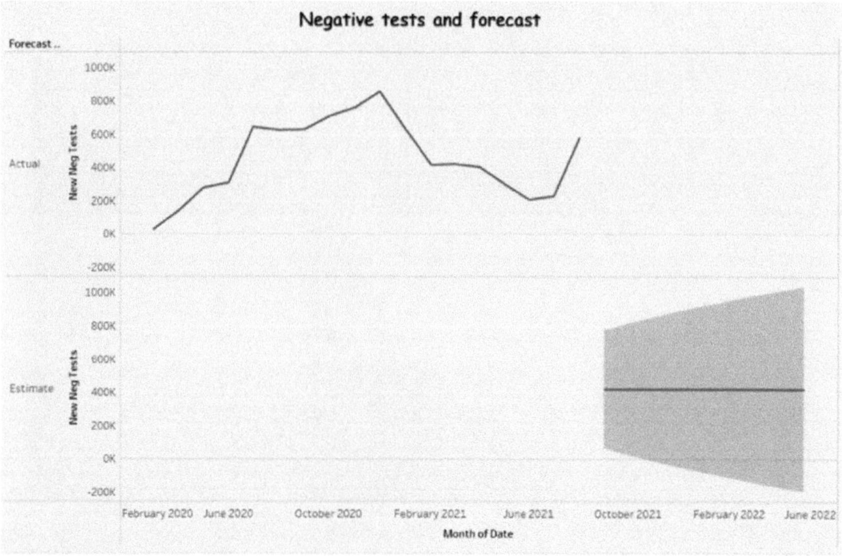

FIGURE 10.11 Forecast of negative tests.

illnesses from a few test result images. It also provides a brief contrast among a couple of CNN architectures, their process and model, about their datasets on which they have been trained, precision, sensitivity, and accuracy they attained. The artificial intelligence software is growing sharply, but also in healthcare [21]. Many unique interdisciplinary pieces of research with unique artificial intelligence and its features suggest the essential and vital gaps of artificial intelligence to assist patients. Continuing to expand artificial intelligence in assisting doctors for a better diagnosis, it is the authors' goal to show the need for educating patients about their disease and supporting the payment system in surgery [8]. Throughout this chapter, the authors constructed three different models of a digital nurse to support patients in booking an appointment, providing them with the test results, and advising them on the time as well as the amount for healthcare payment. The digital multi-task nurse could inform the doctors about their schedule of upcoming appointments and surgeries daily. Finally, this chapter recommended some displays on a mobile platform to provide these models of artificial intelligence [12].

As a conclusion, the researcher states that, by using simple exponential smoothing, the forecast results can be found with the data visualization tool called Tableau. Through much research, it is proven that artificial intelligence and machine learning algorithms are widely used in the implementation of data-driven analytics in various fields, even in the medical and healthcare industry. In this study, a dataset is taken and pre-processed using Tableau to find the plot with the existing data. Through further study, forecast plots are obtained for different parameters such as death rates and negative test cases. With the forecast study, the world can observe COVID-free patients; that is, when the negative test cases increase, the positive test cases will decrease. As an outcome, the patient count will also decrease [1].

KEYWORDS

- **artificial intelligence**
- **data analytics**
- **diagnostics**
- **exponential smoothing**
- **healthcare industry**
- **machine learning**
- **smoothing factor**

REFERENCES

1. Tkachenko, I., Izonin, P., Vitynskyi, N., Lotoshynska, and O. Pavlyuk. (2018). Development of the Non-Iterative Supervised Learning Predictor Based on the Ito Decomposition and SGTM Neural-Like Structure for Managing Medical Insurance Costs. *Data, 3*(4), 1–14.
2. Telenyk, S., Czajkowski, K., Bidiuk, P., & Zharikov, E. (2019). Method of Assessing the State of Monuments based on Fuzzy Logic. In *2019 10th IEEE International Conference on Intelligent Data Acquisition and Advanced Computing Systems: Technology and Applications (IDAACS)* (pp. 500–506). IEEE.
3. Dangare, C. S., & Apte, S. S. (2012). Improved study of heart disease prediction system using data mining classification techniques. *International Journal of Computer Applications, 47*(10), 44–48.
4. Vijiyarani, S., & Sudha, S. (2013). Disease prediction in data mining technique–a survey. *International Journal of Computer Applications & Information Technology, 2*(1), 17–21.

5. Tang, Y., Wang, Y., Cooper, K. M., & Li, L. (2014). Towards big data Bayesian network learning-an ensemble learning based approach. In *2014 IEEE International Congress on Big Data* (pp. 355–357). IEEE.
6. Mulesa P., Perova I. (2015). Fuzzy Spacial Extrapolation Method Using Manhattan Metrics for Tasks of Medical Data Mining. In *Proc. of 12th International Conference on Computer Science and Information Technologies CSIT'2015* (pp. 104–106). Lviv, Ukraine.
7. Bodyanskiy Ye., Perova I., Vynokurova O., Izonin I. (2018). Adaptive Wavelet Diagnostic Neuro-Fuzzy System for Biomedical Tasks. In *Proc. of 14th International Conference on Advanced Trends in Radioelectronics, Telecommunications and Computer Engineering (TCSET)* (pp. 20–24).
8. Perova, O., Litovchenko, Ye., Bodyanskiy, Ye., Brazhnykova, I., Zavgorodnii, P., & Mulesa, P. (2018). Medical Data-Stream Mining in the Area of Electromagnetic Radiation and Low Temperature Influence on Biological Objects. In *Proc. 2018 IEEE Second International Conference on Data Stream Mining & Processing (DSMP)* (pp. 3–6).
9. Perova I., Bodyanskiy Ye., Brazhnykova Ye., & Mulesa P. (2018). Neural Network for Online Principal Component Analysis in Medical Data Mining Tasks. In *IEEE First International Conference on System Analysis & Intelligent Computing (SAIC)* (pp. 150–154).
10. Izonin, I. (2018). The combined use of the Wiener polynomial and SVM for material classification task in medical implants production. *International Journal of Intelligent Systems and Applications, 9*, 40–47.
11. Melnykova, N., Shakhovska, N., & Sviridova, T. (2017). The personalized approach in a medical decentralized diagnostic and treatment. In *2017 14th International Conference the Experience of Designing and Application of CAD Systems in Microelectronics (CADSM)* (pp. 295–297). IEEE.
12. Bai, B. M., Nalini, B. M., & Majumdar, J. (2019). Analysis and detection of diabetes using data mining techniques—a big data application in health care. In *Emerging Research in Computing, Information, Communication and Applications* (pp. 443–455). Springer, Singapore.
13. Dudik, J. M., Kurosu, A., Coyle, J. L., & Sejdić, E. (2015). A comparative analysis of DBSCAN, K-means, and quadratic variation algorithms for automatic identification of swallows from swallowing accelerometry signals. *Computers in Biology and Medicine, 59*, 10–18.
14. Melnykova, N. (2017). Semantic search personalized data as special method of processing medical information. In *Advances in Intelligent Systems and Computing* (pp. 315–325). Springer, Cham.
15. Havens, T. C., & Bezdek, J. C. (2011). An efficient formulation of the improved visual assessment of cluster tendency (iVAT) algorithm. *IEEE Transactions on Knowledge and Data Engineering, 24*(5), 813–822.
16. Hopkins, W., Marshall, S., Batterham, A., & Hanin, J. (2009). Progressive statistics for studies in sports medicine and exercise science. *Medicine+ Science in Sports+ Exercise, 41*(1), 3.
17. Arzubov, M., Shakhovska, N., & Lipinski, P. (2017). Analyzing ways of building user profile based on web surf history. In *2017 12th International Scientific and Technical*

Conference on Computer Sciences and Information Technologies (CSIT) (Vol. 1, pp. 377–380). IEEE.
18. Vidal, M. E., Endris, K. M., Jazashoori, S., Sakor, A., & Rivas, A. (2019). Transforming Heterogeneous Data into Knowledge for Personalized Treatments—A Use Case. *Datenbank-Spektrum, 19*(2), 95–106.
19. Cui, X., Yang, S., & Wang, D. (2016). An algorithm of apriori based on medical big data and cloud computing. In *2016 4th International Conference on Cloud Computing and Intelligence Systems (CCIS)* (pp. 361–365). IEEE.
20. Waring J., et al. (2020). Automated Machine Learning: Review of the State-of-the-Art and Opportunities for Healthcare. *Artificial Intelligence in Medicine, 104*, 101822. DOI.org (Crossref), doi: 10.1016/j.artmed.2020.101822.
21. Kharkovyna, O., (2019). Artificial Intelligence & Deep Learning for Medical Diagnosis. https://www.linkedin.com/pulse/artificial-intelligence-deep-learning-medical-oleksii-kharkovyna/.
22. Ng, Man-Fai, et al. (2020). Predicting the State of Charge and Health of Batteries Using Data-Driven Machine Learning. *Nature Machine Intelligence, 2*(3), 161–170. DOI.org (Crossref), doi:10.1038/s42256-020-0156-7.
23. Rytsar B. (2019). A New Method for Symmetry Recognition in Boolean Functions Based on the Set-Theoretical Logic Differentiation. *Control Systems and Computers, 4*(282), 3–13. DOI.org (Crossref), doi:10.15407/csc.2019.04.003.
24. Lauren Jagus, (2018). "IBM Watson Health: Managing Partnerships to Improve Personalized Medicine," In T. Tucker (Ed.), "*Cases and Tools in Biotechnology Management*," 2018. https://ecampusontario.pressbooks.pub/bio16610w18/chapter/ibm-watson-health-managing-partnerships-to-improve-personalized-medicine/.
25. Kit, S., (2021). Assessing genetic predisposition to cancer for confident decision making.https://www.sophiagenetics.com/wp-content/uploads/2021/09/CEIVD_B.1.3.1.1_r3en_SG_HCS_DS.pdf.
26. Calvanese, D., Calvanese, G., Giacomo, D., Lembo, M., Lenzerini, A., & Poggi, R. (2007). Ontology-based database access. In *Proc. of SEBD–2007* (pp. 324–331).
27. Tkachenko, R., Izonin, I. (2019). Model and Principles for the Implementation of Neural-Like Structures based on Geometric Data Transformations. In Z. B. Hu, & S. Petoukhov (Eds.), *Advances in Computer Science for Engineering and Education. ICCSEEA2018. Advances in Intelligent Systems and Computing, 754* (pp. 578–587). Springer, Cham. https://doi.org/10.1007/978-3-319-91008-6_58.
28. Tkachenko R., Izonin I., Kryvinska K., Chopyak V., Lotoshynska N., Danylyuk D. (2018). Piecewise-linear Approach for Medical Insurance Costs Prediction using SGTM Neural-Like Structure. In N. Shakhovska, S. Montenegro, Ya. Estève, S. Subbotin, N. Kryvinska, I. Izonin (Eds.), *Informatics & Data-Driven Medicine (IDDM 2018). Proceedings of the 1st International Workshop IDDM 2018* (pp. 170–179). CEUR-WS.org.
29. Jaiswal, A., Gianchandani, N., Singh, D., Kumar, V., & Kaur, M. (2020). Classification of the covid-19 infected patients using densenet201 based deep transfer learning. *Journal of Biomolecular Structure and Dynamics, 39*(15), pp. 1–8.
30. Ginat, D. T. (2020). Analysis of head ct scans flagged by deep learning software for acute intracranial hemorrhage. *Neuroradiology, 62*(3), 335–340.

31. Lewick, T., Kumar, M., Hong, R., & Wu, W. (2020). Intracranial hemorrhage detection in ct scans using deep learning. In *2020 IEEE Sixth International Conference on Big Data Computing Service and Applications (BigDataService)* (pp. 169–172). IEEE.
32. Chen, F. C., & Jahanshahi, M. R. (2017). Nb-cnn: Deep learning-based crack detection using convolutional neural network and naïve bayes data fusion. *IEEE Transactions on Industrial Electronics, 65*(5), 4392–4400.
33. Moher, D., Shamseer, L., Clarke, M., Ghersi, D., Liberati, A., Petticrew, M., Shekelle, P., & Stewart, L. A. (2015). Preferred reporting items for systematic review and meta-analysis protocols (prisma-p) 2015 statement. *Systematic Reviews, 4*(1), 1.
34. Liberati, A., Altman, D. G., Tetzlaff, J., Mulrow, C., Gøtzsche, P. C., Ioannidis, J. P., Clarke, M., Devereaux, P. J., Kleijnen, J., & Moher, D. (2009). The prisma statement for reporting systematic reviews and meta-analyses of studies that evaluate health care interventions: explanation and elaboration. *Annals of Internal Medicine, 151*(4), W–65.
35. Elasnaoui, K., & Chawki, Y. (2020). Using x-ray images and deep learning for automated detection of coronavirus disease. *Journal of Biomolecular Structure and Dynamics, 39*(10), 1–22.
36. Holzinger, A., Langs, G., Denk, H., Zatloukal, K., & Müller, H. (2019). Causability and explainability of artificial intelligence in medicine. *Wiley Interdisciplinary Reviews: Data Mining and Knowledge Discovery, 9*(4), e1312.
37. Elazab, N., Soliman, H., El-Sappagh, S., Islam, S., & Elmogy, M. (2020). Objective diagnosis for histopathological images based on machine learning techniques: Classical approaches and new trends. *Mathematics, 8*(11), 1863.
38. Tellez, D., Litjens, G., Bándi, P., Bulten, W., Bokhorst, J.-M., Ciompi, F., & van der Laak, J. (2019). Quantifying the effects of data augmentation and stain color normalization in convolutional neural networks for computational pathology. *Medical Image Analysis, 58*, 101544.
39. Dwivedi, S. A., Borse, R., & Yametkar, A. M. (2014). Lung cancer detection and classification by using machine learning & multinomial bayesian. *IOSR Journal of Electronics and Communication Engineering (IOSRJECE), 9*(1), 69–75.
40. Marsland, S. (2014). *Machine Learning: An Algorithmic Perspective,* Second Edition (2nd ed.). Chapman and Hall/CRC. https://doi.org/10.1201/b17476.
41. Kononenko, I., Bratko, I., & Kukar, M. (1997). Application of machine learning to medical diagnosis. In *Machine Learning and Data Mining: Methods and Applications* (Vol. 389, p. 408).
42. Suzuki, K. (2017). Overview of deep learning in medical imaging. *Radiological Physics and Technology, 10*(3), 257–273.
43. LeCun, Y., Bengio, Y., & Hinton, G. (2015). Deep learning. *Nature, 521*(7553), 436–444.

CHAPTER 11

M-Blockchain: A Futuristic Approach for Healthcare

SHAIK KHAJA MOHIDDIN,[1] BALAGANESH,[2] and MOHAMMED ALI HUSSAIN[3]

[1]*Postdoctoral Fellow, Lincoln University College, Malaysia*

[2]*Professor, Computer Science and Multimedia, Lincoln University College, Malaysia*

[3]*Professor and Associate Dean R&D, KLEF (Deemed to be University), Guntur, Andhra Pradesh, India*

ABSTRACT

Managing data, completing transactions, setting boundaries, and trust building in an open space are all made possible through the innovative use of blockchain technology. A wide range of organizations view blockchain as a significant step forward in cryptography and network security, pointing to applications in widely used computerized money systems like Bitcoin, insight agreements, and smart grids on the Internet of Things. Regardless of the fact that blockchain has gained traction in both the academic and business worlds only recently, the security and assurance of blockchains continue to be the point of convergence of the debate when deploying blockchain in various applications. Distributed systems are becoming more popular thanks to blockchain technology's potential to improve their security and stability. Finance, remote sensing, and data analysis have all benefited from studies using this technique. An appealing characteristic of blockchain technology is that data is immutable and dispersed across

Data-Driven Analytics for Healthcare: Artificial Intelligence and Machine Learning for Medical Diagnostics. Meghna Sharma, Priyanka Vashisht, A. V. Senthil Kumar, Chitra Singh, and Abdelmalek Amine (Eds.)

multiple nodes. This system, on the other hand, is hampered by the danger of a privacy breach due to the sensitive nature of healthcare records. A comprehensive overview of blockchain security and protection is provided in this chapter. Blockchains and their use in Bitcoin-like apps on the online exchanges are first introduced in order to stimulate discussion. As a result, we also depict the fundamental security characteristics that are sustained as the basic demands, erecting obstacles for Bitcoin-like digital money framework, followed by the introduction of additional security and security properties required in several blockchain apps.

11.1 INTRODUCTION

Data on a patient's healthcare is regularly shared among many healthcare providers. During treatment or for medical study, patients are required to submit their data. Medical data is extremely private and must be given explicit authorization in order to be shared or transferred from one organization to another. This consent is required by European and American law. It is difficult for a patient to communicate his or her access control policy in a conventional form of consent. It can be, for example, when a patient desires to acquire an individual perspective about his illness from a different doctor in the same medical facility or prefers not to divulge some of his medical history. Information on an individual's or a population's health status and attributes is the primary focus of health data. Clinical metrics and other essential characteristics, such as behavioral, environmental, and socio-economic data relevant to health and well-being, can now be included with individual or population-based environmental, socio-economic, and behavioral data. Meanwhile, healthcare institutions are gathering data on patients in order to use the information for analytics aimed at promoting, restoring, and maintaining good health for the general public. Additionally, this allows more direct efforts toward improving one's overall health to take place. In recent years, blockchain technology has been widely employed to ensure data security during the digital asset transition process without the involvement of a third party. Patients may be concerned about their privacy and refuse to give their agreement to the collection and use of their data for research purposes. Data anonymization can be a substitute to collect consent. When numerous datasets including anonymized information about a single patient are linked together, the privacy of the patient may be compromised [1]. In the long run, how can we retain track of the information we've communicated about the patient? Because of their medical condition, chronic disease-affected patients or other significant illnesses may have to keep track of their medical history or entrust that responsibility to family members. For most of these patients, keeping track of their medical records, access controls, medications, bills, insurance correspondence, and payments is an inevitable hassle. A patient with cancer, for example, may require immediate knowledge of the radiation dose received over the course of the patient's lifetime of treatment. An essential treatment could be delayed due to issues with permission management and data transfer. While blockchain is a relatively new technology, it's quickly gaining traction from businesses, academics, and the government. Because of its unique features, blockchain is now considered a cutting-edge technology that may be used to address complex problems in a wide range of exciting new applications. Blockchain technology has the potential to change a broad range of fields, including finance, healthcare, and education. Due to its fault tolerance, traceability, scalability, and high security, blockchain has great promise for use in the healthcare industry. By conducting in-depth investigations, the benefits, obstacles, and important use cases for implementing blockchain in the health industry are presented to the general public. With the expansion of IT in healthcare over the last two decades, a new threat has emerged with concerns about security, privacy, and ethical considerations for patient data [2]. Data mining of patient health records is an important part of digital health, but it is also recognized as a serious security risk. Threats to patients' privacy and their ability to lead normal lives include intrusions into their private lives and life-altering events planned behind their backs without their knowledge.

Computer science, for example, can make a substantial contribution in this area because the healthcare industry requires more help from other professions [3]. A few examples include, but are not limited to, the maintenance of electronic health records, the development of tools to aid in disease diagnosis, the genetic prediction of genomes, and many more. There is a lot of patient data being stored in public and private health organizations every day, and this poses the question of how to deal with it all. This difficulty has been solved in recent years by using a common idea such as BDA which may be characterized as a set of novel methodologies employed in enormous datasets of high complexity, in which typical architectures cannot be supported [4]. Healthcare diagnostics, other applications along with magnetic resonance imaging, could get advantage from the use of Big Data. As a diverse field, computing is a useful tool for enhancing and automating processes in a variety of fields. A variety of medical issues can be solved with the help of computing's array of tools. It has the potential to increase healthcare systems' quality, efficiency, and cost-savings [5].

11.2 BLOCKCHAIN

There are various uses for Bitcoin Blockchain technology in finance, trading, telecommunications, and manufacturing. The technology is called Blockchain. In 2008, this technology was first introduced. A group of people operating under the pseudonym Satoshi Nakamoto came up with the idea. When it comes to market capitalization, Bitcoin is a virtual currency that has taken off. As its name suggests, blockchain is a network of linked blocks, but its significance goes well beyond that. Information stored digitally in a public database (the "block") is the context of the words "block" and "chain." Constraints such as intermittent unreliability or non-existent nodes might lead to data inconsistencies in a dispersed database model. The main distinction between traditional distributed databases and blockchains is their ability to deal with conflicts. Consensus, or resolving conflicts, is a primary function of blockchains. While blockchain technology is an online version of a physical blockchain, it provides businesses with the ability to store and securely track their financial transactions. Contact between the organization and the P2P network can only be established if this field is checked, as the ledger gets encrypted during this process. In a word, the blockchain is a transparent, reliable, and decentralized ledger constructed on a peer-to-peer network. While Bitcoin is still the most talked-about cryptocurrency, experts have been promoting blockchain-based applications as well. In the blockchain network, decentralization means that the blockchain is dispersed among a network of nodes. With the ability to make, validate, and authenticate a new transaction that will be recorded in the blockchain, each node may verify the activity of other nodes in the network. This decentralized architecture, with its tamper resistance and lack of single-point failure risks, ensures robust and secure blockchain operations. Although various distributed frameworks are based on agreement and following qualities, blockchain is unique (Table 11.1).

TABLE 11.1 Blockchain Properties

Property	Description
Censorship safe	As a decentralized network with no central authority, the blockchain allows for open communication and execution by anybody. You can't go back and adjust an exchange that has already been confirmed. In addition to the previously indicated legal justifications, blockchain innovation contains four key components [6].
Consensus	As a part of the Proof of Work (PoW) standard, it is essential to ensure that no single excavator hub has control over the entire blockchain system and that the exchange history is maintained.
Cryptography	It ensures that the system's data is protected with strong cryptographic encryption. It only allows data to be decrypted by those who have been approved. Only those who have been granted access to the data can decrypt it.
Ledger	Almost every transaction that takes place within the system is recorded in this central database, which can be accessed by anyone using the system. As a rule, once data is saved, it cannot be wiped out by any methods whatsoever. It ensures that each transaction is thoroughly vetted and then accepted by the majority of clients at a given point in time [7].
Permission less	A person's ability to work within the system is unrestricted; no consent is required.
Smart contracts	It is used to authorize and authorize the system's members.
Trust less	The components of the system are incomprehensible to one another. They can, however, coordinate, communicate, and function together being aware of each other, implying that no sophisticated character is required to carry out any transactions between the substances.

To collect and track resources without the need for a centralized authority, a blockchain acts as a widely diffused, safe, and secure ledger. Instead of a single concentrated authority making all the decisions, a P2P network where consensus is reached by a majority of authorities rather than a single authority allows two parties to interact and share resources [8]. Invaders who try to take control of the system by compromising the central commander are basically safe. There is a lot of interest in blockchain technology from both industry and academia. This technique has lately been used to expand a number of popular and active networking research projects. These applications include IoT [9], cloud storage [10], and healthcare [11]. Overall, the technology has proven its worth in every application that requires a centralized ledger in recent times. Some of the blockchain network's uses include network management and security services such as secrecy, authenticity, confidentiality, and verification. Third-party authenticated or verifiable services are used for these services, which concludes that security is a significant concern for current apps. On the other side, the blockchain's guarantee of security solves several conventional difficulties, including providing a completely distributed, consensus-based, and practical solution. Figure 11.1 illustrates the differences between traditional access monitoring and blockchain-based access monitoring.

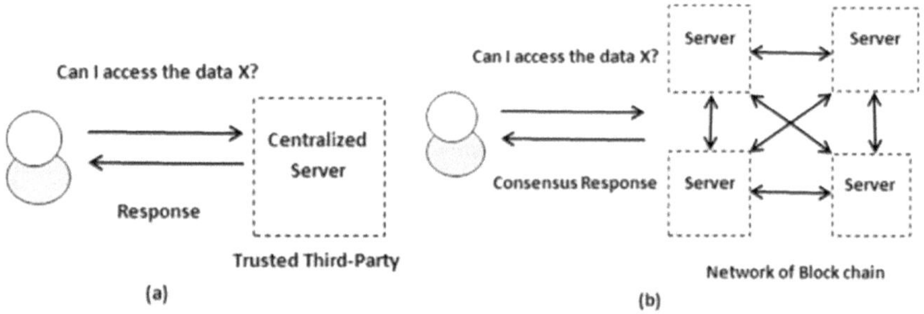

FIGURE 11.1 (a) Conventional centralized access control; and (b) blockchain-based access control.

Source: Adapted from Ref. [42]

Rather than relying on a single, central authority, Blockchain technology allows for secure and "trustless" transactions directly among the parties involved. It uses encryption and game theory to provide decentralization, immutability, and consensus. DApps and cryptocurrencies are just two of the many applications of this technology. It is now possible to control the exchange or redistribution of digital assets among two or more parties according to rules or arrangements previously developed between the involved participants using smart contracts, which are advancements in Blockchain tech as implemented in Ethereum's blockchain. Blockchain-assisted creation of DApps is made possible by smart contracts, which may store data objects and define activities on the data. Healthcare can benefit from smart contracts by creating safe and effective technological infrastructures that increase care coordination and quality, and consequently the well-being of individuals and communities. In an ideal world, software applications and web-based services would coexist.

11.3 PATIENT MONITORING

Sensor security must be improved since IoT and sensors are used in a wide range of settings, including medical facilities such as hospitals, clinics, and other healthcare facilities [12]. Smart bracelets or other gadgets that can be placed on patients are the sensors. When tracking patients, personal and sensitive data is collected by sensors. Blockchain can assist in enhancing the safety of these devices. Regulations such as Brazil's LGPD [13], Europe's GDPR [14], and the United States' HIPAA [15] must be followed to secure personal information. Systems must protect patients' personal information, and blockchain technology can help by protecting the privacy of healthcare data. A number of new technologies have emerged to enhance and strengthen traditional systems in the workplace.

These new technologies include the IoT, sensor networks, and wearable electronics. The usage of Wireless Body Area Networks (WBANs) in medicine is one example of how technological advancements can improve the medical field. Personal networks that include sensors implanted or wearable, as well as a central unit for data transit, can benefit from this idea [16]. WBAN networks for patient monitoring using blockchain are shown in Figure 11.2 [17].

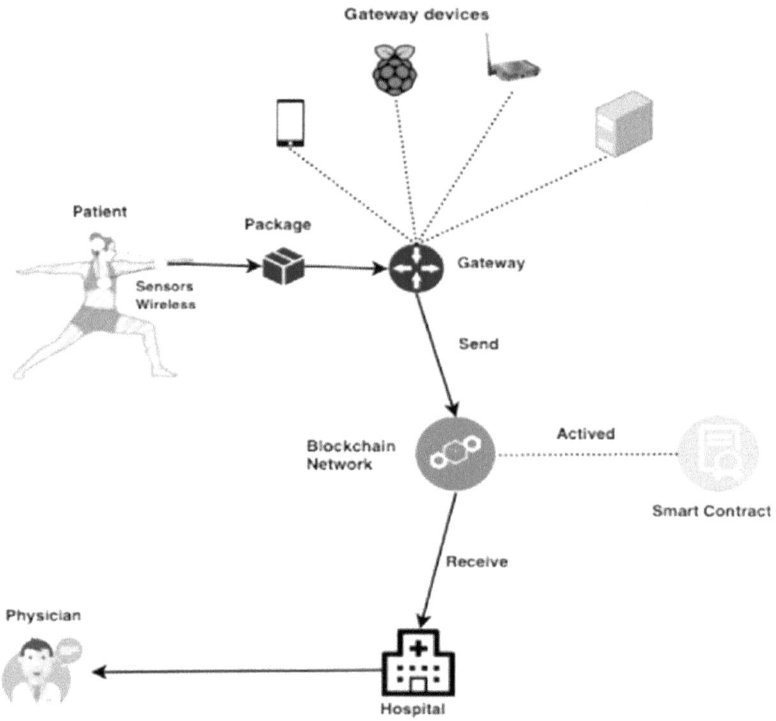

FIGURE 11.2 WBANs for patient monitoring.

Source: Adapted from Ref. [43]

Keeping track of a patient's progress is a vital part of the healthcare system because it aids in the obey of the patient's therapy. Wearable device technologies and gateways, as well as WBANS protocols and protocols, can enhance monitoring quality. The capacity to send patient data over a secure communication channel has several drawbacks, including a lack of consistency and reliability [18]. However, other new technologies, such as blockchain, may assist in solving these issues. Due to characteristics like irreversibility and data privacy that it incorporates, this technology can improve the security of information transit. Blockchain can help with patient monitoring by developing structures that increase the reliability of the process based on the characteristics listed above. In their study, Linn & Koo [19] describe a blockchain-based architecture for the exchange of sensor-based health data that boasts all the benefits that blockchain has to offer. When sensors like a cardiac monitor and others are combined, a patient will still have control over the data they produce. An information repository based on blockchain technology is proposed by the authors. This can be used for a variety of healthcare-related research reasons. The data generated aids in patient follow-up and may possibly speed up the identification and management of illness. Uddin, et al. [20] is yet another example of how blockchain technology might be used to monitor patients. They research the use of personal sensor networks for remote patient monitoring. Additionally, this system makes use of blockchain technology to move sensor-generated data up and down the proposed architecture's hierarchical chain. If you don't have to rely on a trustworthy third party, this technique reduces communication overhead. It also provides transparency and immutability [21, 22].

11.4 VALIDATION PROCESSING BLOCK CHAIN

Mining is another term for the blockchain validation process that is used by certain algorithms, such as proof-of-work [23]. Consensus algorithms are commonly used to carry out this procedure, which also determines the rules by which nodes validate blocks. To ensure that all nodes contributing to validation receive a suitable response, the consensus protocol follows the track in order to carry out the transactions. Because of this, they are in charge of deciding whether or not the block gets added to the chain. Consensus techniques have been developed to improve the reliability of the blockchain's block validation network. Tables 11.2 and 11.3 gives the most common blockchain healthcare protocols that have been outlined in the literature.

TABLE 11.2 Blockchain Protocols

Protocol	Description
PoW	A cryptographic problem is solved by the nodes complicated in the validation process. The right to construct a new block which gears a transaction is granted to the node that finds a solution first. Another point to consider is that some PoW implementations, like Bitcoin, pay out a reward to the algorithm's winner.
PoS	The validations are chosen based on the number of network members. As a result, the more coins it has, the more likely it is that it will be required to verify blocks, and as a result, this node will evaluate whether or not block is genuine.
PBFT	Client and server nodes make up this system. There are three stages to the PBFT validation process: • The client node needs to send an application to server node; • The server nodes communicate the operation to certain other server nodes, which decide whether it is genuine or not; • If a server node accepts the transaction, it sends a readiness message to the other nodes. A high number of nodes should approve a transaction in order for it to be on "confirmation alert;" • To prove its action, each authorized node transmits a digital connection to the network; • The node that sent the action receives the response, regardless of whether it was confirmed or not.

TABLE 11.3 Survey on Blockchain Protocols

Protocol	Survey Outcomes
PoW	Securely transferring medical records, maintaining patient confidentiality, and making the process as simple as possible [24–26].
PoS	Distributing medical images [27].
PBFT	Health information exchanges *via* med tokens are safe and secure and allow for the auditing of access logs to medical records, as well as the sharing of healthcare records [28–30].

11.5 BLOCKCHAIN LIMITATIONS

It's not always easy to manage who has access to what parts of a cloud security system. Planning and thinking about how to deal with hundreds of people accessing systems from all over the world and using a variety of devices can be a difficult endeavor. Hackers of all shades will have an easier time exploiting systems with several layers of security. You can understand how a broken chain, or a weak link, can cause chaos at any level by looking at Figure 11.1. There is an increasing number of devices competing for speedy and secure access to data in a scattered environment like ours. Cloud computing enables on-demand delivery of a wide range of computer services over the internet. Most of the time, we only pay for what we actually use when we utilize a service. Keeping up with the demands of an ever-expanding business like IT is a difficult undertaking. When on-premises resources are insufficient, cloud service providers' enticing characteristics must be taken advantage of. Some common examples of cloud computing services include virtualization, software as a service, and the underlying hardware and software of the cloud environment (IaaS). Customers are all different, thus no single cloud can suit their requirements. For the first time, cloud technologies that are entirely decentralized can be established thanks to smart contracts or blockchain. Many people also propose using decentralized cloud alternatives that are fully integrated and allow large vendors to meet all of these demands. Large organizations all around the world are using virtual servers to host their websites. In one section of the world, users and staff have access to systems that are situated elsewhere. Depending on the time of day or the amount of demand in a particular region of the world, servers might be moved from one data center to another (Table 11.4).

TABLE 11.4 Blockchain Limitations

Limitation	Description
Throughput	For every rise in the number of transactions, a greater number of network nodes must be checked, which might lead to a slowdown in the overall network. When dealing with healthcare systems, high throughput can be a concern because a diagnosis that could save a life can be hampered if there is no quick access.
Latency	If a successful attack occurs during the 10-minute validation period, it could have a negative impact on the security of the system. The dynamic nature of healthcare systems needs constant access, since any delay might have a negative impact on exam analysis.
Security	This can be hacked if an entity gets control of 51% of the network's computing capabilities. A weakened health system can lead to a lack of faith in healthcare providers, which is a crucial concern.
Resource consumption	The mining process uses a significant amount of energy, which could result in a significant loss of resources. The number of devices required to keep tabs on patients in a healthcare setting means that energy consumption is significant; yet the usage of the blockchain could potentially result in high processing and energy expenditures. Handling these costs can be a challenge for corporations.

TABLE 11.4 *(Continued)*

Limitation	Description
Usability	Because these technologies are so difficult to use, usability is also a concern. In addition, a user-friendly API must be created for API users. The systems should be simple and intuitive because health practitioners lack the same level of technical expertise as IT specialists.
Centralization	There are several techniques to mining that incline to centralize the miners and, as a consequence, this decreases the network's ability to function reliably. It is possible for hostile attacks to gain access to the data stored in this susceptible central node.
Privacy	The Bitcoin framework is widely regarded to be able to secure the privacy of blockchain's nodes. However, the findings of Zheng et al. [31] disprove this premise. In addition, blockchain-based systems require strategies to make this capability available. Compliance with the G is required for blockchain-based solutions. Because of privacy rules and regulations, blockchain-based technologies are required to comply with the GDPR.
Scalability and IoT overhead	Scalability and additional processing resources in an IoT setting are two other drawbacks to the blockchain system. As the number of people using a blockchain system grows, so does the computational load on the blockchain infrastructure as a whole, making scalability an issue [32]. When there are a large number of special devices or sensors, it becomes more challenging since their processing power is significantly lower than that of a typical computer, transferring much of the required materials to other processors like a network edge or the cloud [33].
Key management	Cryptographic techniques using private and public keys are required to secure data kept on the blockchain ledger [34]. As with any other system capable of storing information, blockchain technology must have security and privacy measures in place. All participants store blockchain data; most cryptographic operations necessitate the usage of keys in order to enable certain cryptographic processes. Current important management techniques are not suitable for blockchain since a single key for all blocks is insecure, and if the key is compromised, all data would be released, making the system vulnerable. To save and recover the (considerably) huge numbers of individual blocks' unique keys, a one-key-per-block approach would be impractical.
Lack of standardization	An immature technology like blockchain is hampered by a lack of standardization and hence development [35]. For example, governments around the world are exploring implementing the use of blockchain technology in areas such as voting [33]. Countries like Estonia are considering e-residency, which is the process of creating an online account to verify a citizen's residency in a given state and allowing them to vote using that account [37]. The use of blockchain technology in tax and social contexts has also been investigated by other scholars [38]. There must be a high degree of standardization among the numerous parties involved if all of these different infrastructure and application types are to be made possible. The issue of uniformity and regulations will only become more critical as more governments turn to blockchain as a solution.

TABLE 11.4 *(Continued)*

Limitation	Description
Blockchain specific vulnerabilities	The implementation and architecture of the blockchain system itself introduces a number of risks that are not present in other distributed ledger technologies. Block withholding, 51% attack, eclipse attack, selfish mining, double-spending, and block discarding are all examples of blockchain-specific vulnerabilities that can be exploited by attackers [39]. In order to construct a protected environment, blockchain relies on a consensus method in which miners or a group of legitimate participants certifies each transaction on any digital asset. As a result of this, miners typically require some incentive to complete the authentication process, which is usually the solution to some sort of cryptographic equation [40].
Decentralized storage and privacy leakage	Blockchain systems' decentralized storage is a fundamental differentiator, allowing users to post data across multiple services without relying on a single source [41]. Since a user must access the public ledger, which is spread over the blockchain, a major drawback of a decentralized system is the risk of data leakage into the open public domain. In order to decrypt a user's data, the user must enter a private key, which could potentially expose the user's sensitive information. The public key must be on the network at the time of verification and decryption because the data is not stored locally, which is unlike a centralized database. Healthcare facilities face particular challenges because of the high standards they must meet.
General software vulnerabilities	There are also general software flaws that can be exploited in order to carry out hostile attacks on the blockchain. Identity fraud and data exfiltration can then be facilitated by these hostile attacks [36]. When a hostile actor obtains access to a blockchain patient's private key, they acquire knowledge of everything the target has ever disclosed on the blockchain, culminating in identity theft. Illegal behavior such as illicit firearms, drugs, and other commodities can be sold discreetly via the distributed ledger. The deployment of double-spending of cryptocurrencies can also be made possible by hacking into poorly maintained blockchain software, such as a bitcoin exchange [36].

11.6 CONCLUSION

The blockchain community has taken a keen interest in the technological problem of scaling blockchain to handle high volumes of clinical transactions. Some of the problems that the healthcare business has could be solved with blockchain technology. Integrity, security, decentralization, authentication, and availability principles owing to the block-related and global infrastructure represent the strongest potential of blockchain technology in the healthcare sector. As the IoT, smart gadgets, and sensing devices proliferate, the healthcare industry is scrambling to keep up. There are many advantages to using such technology in the healthcare industry, but there are also many disadvantages. For example, hostile actors can access and copy the data, making it difficult to communicate records between hospitals. Health difficulties or misdiagnosis may ensue, as well as a difficulty in authenticating a patient's identification, as a result of this. Patient-centered interoperability presents a wide range of difficulties, including those related to patient consent, administration, privacy, and security. The use of blockchain technology to create a safe platform for data exchange offers a promising solution to these problems. Consideration of privacy and security issues, such as the anonymous-but-not-private element of most blockchain implementations, as well as concerns around patient key services and clinical interaction, will also be necessary. Patient-facing data interfaces will need incentives to encourage interoperability, and this will be a constant challenge. These issues must be addressed in the future. Designing a patient-centric paradigm that is both usable and beneficial while also aligning incentives with many stakeholders will be critical in this regard. Managing data permission and storage standards will need more clarity as the GDPR is implemented throughout the EU and other privacy laws are revised in other jurisdictions.

KEYWORDS

- **blockchain**
- **decentralized apps**
- **general data protection regulation**
- **practical byzantine fault tolerance**
- **proof of stake**
- **proof of work**
- **wireless body area networks**

REFERENCES

1. Baig, M. M., Sweeney, P. T., Caverlee, J., Giles, C. L., Zhan, J., & Tsioutsiouliklis, K. (2011). Cloning for privacy protection in multiple independent data publications. In *Proceedings of the 20th ACM international Conference on Information and Knowledge Management* (pp. 2015–2024). ACM.

2. Mammadova, M. (2015). The problems of information security of electronic personal health data. In *2015 7th International Conference on Information Technology in Medicine and Education (ITME)* (pp. 678–682). IEEE.
3. Wechsler, R., Santos, L. F., Junqueira, M. F., Wietzikoski, E. C., & Martins, J. R. (2003). A informática no consultório médico. *Jornal de Pediatria, 79*(S3), S3-S12.
4. Lee, C. H., & Yoon, H. J. (2017). Medical big data: promise and challenges. *Kidney Research and Clinical Practice, 36*(1), 3–11.
5. Chaudhry, B., Wang, J., Wu, S., Maglione, M., Mojica, W., Roth, E., & Shekelle, P. G. (2006). Systematic review: impact of health information technology on quality, efficiency, and costs of medical care. *Annals of Internal Medicine, 144*(10), 742–752.
6. Singh, M., Singh, A., & Kim, S. (2018). Blockchain: A game changer for securing IoT data. In *2018 IEEE 4th World Forum on Internet of Things (WF-IoT)* (pp. 51–56). IEEE.
7. Bhushan, B., Gupta, S., Pathak, V. K., & Singh, V. (2021). Unification of Blockchain and Internet of Things (BIoT): requirements, working model, challenges and future directions. *Wireless Networks, 27*(1), 55–90.
8. Christidis, K., & Devetsikiotis, M. (2016). Blockchains and smart contracts for the internet of things. *IEEE Access, 4*, 2292–2303.
9. Arora, A., Kaur, A., Bhushan, B., & Saini, H. (2019, July). Security concerns and future trends of internet of things. In *2019 2nd International Conference on Intelligent Computing, Instrumentation and Control Technologies (ICICICT)* (Vol. 1, pp. 891–896). IEEE.
10. Zhang, Y., Xu, C., Lin, X., & Shen, X. S. (2019). Blockchain-based public integrity verification for cloud storage against procrastinating auditors. *IEEE Transactions on Cloud Computing, 9*(3), 923–937.
11. Mettler, M. (2016). Blockchain technology in healthcare: The revolution starts here. In *2016 IEEE 18th International Conference on e-Health Networking, Applications and Services (Healthcom)* (pp. 1–3). IEEE.
12. Cha, S. C., Chen, P. C., Su, S. Y., & Yeh, C. W. (2018). A blockchain connected gateway for BLE-based devices in the internet of things. *IEEE Access, 6*, 24639–24649.
13. Mulholland, C. S. (2018). Dados pessoais sensíveis e a tutela de direitos fundamentais: uma análise à luz da Lei Geral de Proteção de Dados (Lei 13.709/18). *Revista de Direitos e Garantias Fundamentais, 19*(3), 159–180.
14. Philipp, A. J. (2016). How the GDPR will change the world. *European Data Protection Law Review (EDPL), 3*, 287–289.
15. Office for Civil Rights. (2003). Summary of the HIPAA privacy rule. *HIPAA Compliance Assistance*.
16. Ali, A., & Khan, F. A. (2015). Key agreement schemes in wireless body area networks: Taxonomy and state-of-the-art. *Journal of Medical Systems, 39*(10), 1–14.
17. Salem, O., Su, S., Abbes, T., Obaidat, M. S., & Jamalipour, A. (2014). Online anomaly detection in wireless body area networks for reliable healthcare monitoring. *IEEE Journal of Biomedical and Health Informatics, 18*(5), 1541–1551.
18. Ren, Y., Werner, J. P., Meinel, C., & Liscano, R. (2010). Monitoring patients via a secure and mobile healthcare system. *IEEE Wireless Communications, 17*(1), 59–65.
19. Linn, L. A., & Koo, M. B. (2016). Blockchain for health data and its potential use in health IT and health care related research. In ONC/NIST Use of Blockchain for

Healthcare and Research Workshop. Gaithersburg, Maryland, United States: ONC/NIST (pp. 1–10).
20. Uddin, M. A., Stranieri, A., Gondal, I., & Balasubramanian, V. (2018). Continuous patient monitoring with a patient centric agent: A block architecture. *IEEE Access, 6*, 32700–32726.
21. Halamka, J. D., Lippman, A., & Ekblaw, A. (2017). The potential for blockchain to transform electronic health records. *Harvard Business Review, 3*(3), 2–5.
22. Stagnaro, C. (2017). White paper: Innovative blockchain uses in health care. *Freed Associates, 28,* 2018, https://www.freedassociates.com/wpcontent/uploads/2017/08/Blockchain_White_Paper.pdf.
23. Nakamoto, S. (2008). Bitcoin: A peer-to-peer electronic cash system. *Decentralized Business Review*, 21260.
24. Azaria, A., Ekblaw, A., Vieira, T., & Lippman, A. (2016). Medrec: Using blockchain for medical data access and permission management. In *2016 2nd International Conference on Open and Big Data (OBD)* (pp. 25–30). IEEE.
25. da Conceição, A. F., Albuquerque, V. H. C., Cortez, P. C., & Filho, J. G. P. (2018). Electronic health records using blockchain technology. arXiv preprint arXiv:1804.10078. 2018 April 26.
26. Guo, R., Shi, H., Zhao, Q., & Zheng, D. (2018). Secure attribute-based signature scheme with multiple authorities for blockchain in electronic health records systems. *IEEE Access, 6*, 11676–11686.
27. Patel, V. (2019). A framework for secure and decentralized sharing of medical imaging data via blockchain consensus. *Health Informatics Journal, 25*(4), 1398–1411.
28. Anderson, J. (2018). Securing, standardizing, and simplifying electronic health record audit logs through permissioned blockchain technology. *Dartmouth College Undergraduate Theses*. 135).
29. Dubovitskaya, A., Xu, Z., Ryu, S., Schumacher, M., & Wang, F. (2017). Secure and trustable electronic medical records sharing using blockchain. In *AMIA Annual Symposium Proceedings* (Vol. 2017, p. 650). American Medical Informatics Association.
30. Praveen, G., Singh, P. K., & Ranjan, P. (2021). The impact of blockchain on the healthcare environment. *Journal of Informatics Electrical and Electronics Engineering (JIEEE), 2*(2), 1–11.
31. Zheng, Z., Xie, S., Dai, H., Chen, X., & Wang, H. (2018). Blockchain challenges and opportunities: A survey. *International Journal of Web and Grid Services, 14*(4), 352–375.
32. Roehrs, A., Da Costa, C. A., & Righi, R. D. R. (2017). OmniPHR: A distributed architecture model to integrate personal health records. *Journal of Biomedical Informatics, 71*, 70–81.
33. Hou, H. (2017). The application of blockchain technology in E-government in China. In *2017 26th International Conference on Computer Communication and Networks (ICCCN)* (pp. 1–4). IEEE.
34. Zhao, H., Zhang, Y., Xu, Y., & Xie, W. (2017). Lightweight backup and efficient recovery scheme for health blockchain keys. In *2017 IEEE 13th International Symposium on Autonomous Decentralized System (ISADS)* (pp. 229–234). IEEE.

35. Ølnes, S., Ubacht, J., & Janssen, M. (2017). Blockchain in government: Benefits and implications of distributed ledger technology for information sharing. *Government Information Quarterly, 34*(3), 355–364.
36. Jiang, P., Chen, H., Zhang, L., Guo, S., & Lu, Z. (2020). Searchain: Blockchain-based private keyword search in decentralized storage. *Future Generation Computer Systems, 107*, 781–792.
37. Sullivan, C., & Burger, E. (2017). E-residency and blockchain. *Computer Law & Security Review, 33*(4), 470–481.
38. Pokrovskaia, N. N. (2017). Tax, financial and social regulatory mechanisms within the knowledge-driven economy: Blockchain algorithms and fog computing for the efficient regulation. In *2017 XX IEEE International Conference on Soft Computing and Measurements (SCM)* (pp. 1–4). IEEE.
39. Xu, J. J. (2016). Are blockchains immune to all malicious attacks? *Financial Innovation, 2*(1), 1–9.
40. Tosh, D. K., Shetty, S., Liang, X., Kamhoua, C. A., & Njilla, L. (2017). Security implications of blockchain cloud with analysis of block withholding attack. In *2017 17th IEEE/ACM International Symposium on Cluster, Cloud and Grid Computing (CCGRID)* (pp. 458–467). IEEE.
41. Liang, X., Shetty, S., Tosh, D. K., Kamhoua, C., Kwiat, K., & Njilla, L. (2017). Provchain: A blockchain-based data provenance architecture in cloud environment with enhanced privacy and availability. In *2017 17th IEEE/ACM International Symposium on Cluster, Cloud and Grid Computing (CCGRID)* (pp. 468–477). IEEE.
42. Ghaffari, Fariba, et al. "A novel access control method via smart contracts for internet-based service provisioning." IEEE Access 9 (2021): 81253-81273
43. Xu, Xiaoling, et al. "A survey on energy harvesting and integrated data sharing in wireless body area networks." (2015).

CHAPTER 12

Blockchain in Healthcare: Evolution, Applications, and Challenges

SHAIK RASOOL,[1] UMA N. DULHARE,[2] and A. V. SENTHIL KUMAR[3]

[1]*Methodist College of Engineering and Technology, Hyderabad, Telangana, India*

[2]*Muffakham Jah College of Engineering and Technology, Hyderabad, Telangana, India*

[3]*Hindusthan College of Arts and Science, Coimbatore, Tamil Nadu, India*

ABSTRACT

Blockchain is providing a safe and secure environment for online transactions that has amazed the world. It is estimated that this technology will be adopted by almost all companies around the world in various domains due to its numerous benefits. Therefore, it is essential to understand and comprehend how the evolution has started and the road to the future. Every aspect of blockchain starts from its components and types, supporting the understanding of the mechanism involved in blockchain. For implementation, it is critical to choose the right blockchain technology for adaptation. Deploying blockchain technology requires multidisciplinary knowledge and various advantages that it provides. The security provided by blockchain is the core of the entire system that has attracted and gained focus from all industries for its rapid adoption. Thus, learning all these becomes integral for an individual or company looking for solutions provided by blockchain.

Data-Driven Analytics for Healthcare: Artificial Intelligence and Machine Learning for Medical Diagnostics. Meghna Sharma, Priyanka Vashisht, A. V. Senthil Kumar, Chitra Singh, and Abdelmalek Amine (Eds.)

12.1 INTRODUCTION TO BLOCKCHAIN

With the increase in technological advancements in this era, smart devices and intelligent systems that are smart enough to efficiently link, communicate, and complete the required tasks are needed [1]. Blockchain refers to technology that provides a solution to everyone's ancient beliefs. It appeared on the market using the infamous Bitcoin cryptocurrency. It provides a graphic design that allows us to rely on distribution (Internet or Web) without disturbing anyone in it. It runs a friends and acquaintance website and has its own copy of the transaction. This helps to avoid arbitrators, and then the entire transaction process is completed with the machine protocol. A record is set among the many entities that everyone can visit but nothing can stop it. An encrypted, secure distributed website stores data about each transaction from the start.

12.1.1 KEY ELEMENTS OF THE BLOCKCHAIN

The information in the blockchain is stored in encrypted segments called blocks. The next block contains information about the first block and creates a chain called the Blockchain. Blockchain privacy is maintained with complex cryptographic hashes and public key encryption, which help achieve transparency. It adds new business to existing knowledge based on the unity of miners involved in the network. Trade guarantee rules are marked about algorithms and implemented by the miners who also receive certificates, commodity certificates, and other foundations of existing economic assets on site [2].

The ledger runs on a peer-to-peer network, so any boss who interferes with the network will receive a copy of the original. Now, as a matter of fact, every node on the website is owned by a person and a server. Figure 12.1 summarizes the key elements of the blockchain. The server or user will be one of them. The node can start working, which is the smallest block in the entire chain. Blocks are assembled to form a block, but this block is added to the chain after being mined by miners or certified nodes. Administrative authorities set different rules for blockchain management [3].

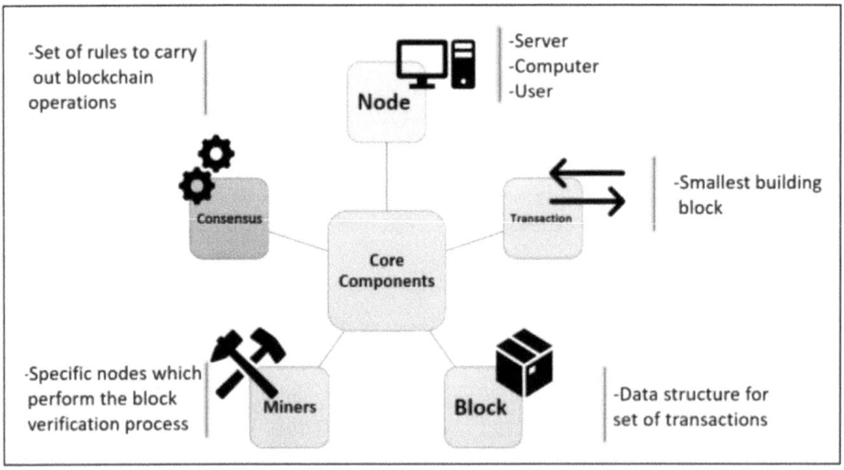

FIGURE 12.1 The core of the blockchain.

12.2 EVOLUTION OF BLOCKCHAIN IN THE MODERN ERA

The development of Blockchain for finance began. It is now emerging from cryptocurrency and could have a huge impact on many businesses. Its main purpose is to eliminate third-party money changers by creating digital products. A blockchain is a digital ledger that captures the entire history of online transactions. A combination of interconnected networks has a unique hash based on time. All blockchain information is persistent and cannot be changed. Figure 12.2 shows a simplified version of the blockchain. The first block of this chain is called the genesis block. All these chains contain all the data and are linked to a point beyond their past.

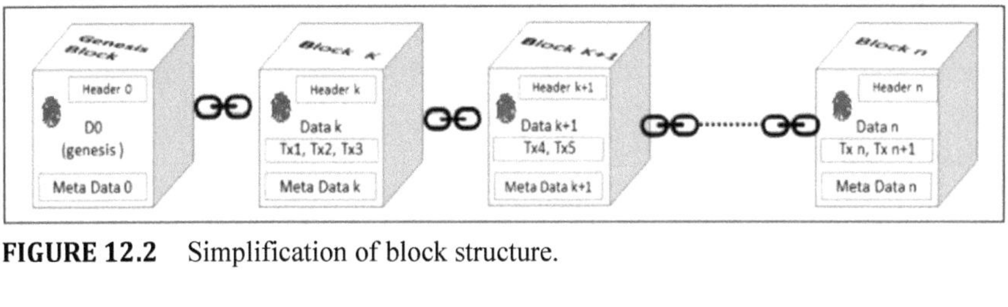

FIGURE 12.2 Simplification of block structure.

A block that defines a block and all its content, like a human finger, is always different. When you block, its hash value is calculated. Changing the content of the block will make the hash value different. Each block also has a hash of the first block. It is an effective pulley design. Blockchain is a distributed architecture so there is no central authorization. Each blockchain node receives a complete copy of the entire chain, so the node uses this copy to verify that everything is OK. Each block has a fixed duration, so it is virtually impossible to interact with the data. When a new block is created, it is sent to each chain. Each node will be checked if the block is not received, and a consensus is reached. Blockchain has no root, so it does a good job.

12.3 THE MAJOR ELEMENTS OF BLOCKCHAIN TECHNOLOGY

Major elements of Blockchain technology can be the following three elements (Figure 12.3):

- Decentralization;
- Transparency; and
- Immutability.

12.3.1 DECENTRALIZATION

Decentralization implies the transfer of control and authorization from a centralized entity to a distributed network. In a distributed network, organizations are extremely careful to ease the intensity of trust that applicants must put on each other and influence their competence to implement authority or control alone in ways that affect network activity [4]. When developing a solution, the three key elements in the construction industry are: determining, classifying, and subdividing. While blockchain technology often uses a distributed network, the blockchain functions themselves cannot be categorized as decentralized or not. Instead, the classification is insignificant and ought to be applied to all kinds of blockchain applications. By distributing supervision and accessing assets in one application, you can achieve increasingly fair services. Managing distribution often requires industry improvements, such as lower costs, but preferably the replacement necessary to improve the security and level of services they create.

12.3.1.1 FRUITFULNESS OF DECENTRALIZATION

1. **Offers a Trust Less Ecosystem:** Provides a reliable environment in mixed blockchain management, anonymous or trusted by others. Each site member obtains a version of the identical information in the form of book distribution. If an associate's ledger is misrepresented or corrupted in any way, most members of the network will reject it.

2. **Improves Data Appeasement:** Most companies exchange data with partners. On the other hand, this information is usually duplicated and stored on each page of information and is only updated when new lines are needed. Each time the file is duplicated, it can result in lost or inaccurate data at work. By keeping personal information confidential, all organizations can access and share personal information in real time.

3. **Diminishes Vulnerability:** Decentralization can reduce the levels of vulnerability in a system that is highly dependent on certain entities. These obvious weaknesses can cause system breakdowns, including failure to deliver on promises or enhance service efficacy due to insufficient assets, short lead times, congestion, lack of motivation for quality assistance, or exploitation.

4. **Elevates Asset Allocation:** Improving equipment distribution transportation services can help enhance equipment distribution so that service commitment can be more efficient and stable, with a decrease in failure.

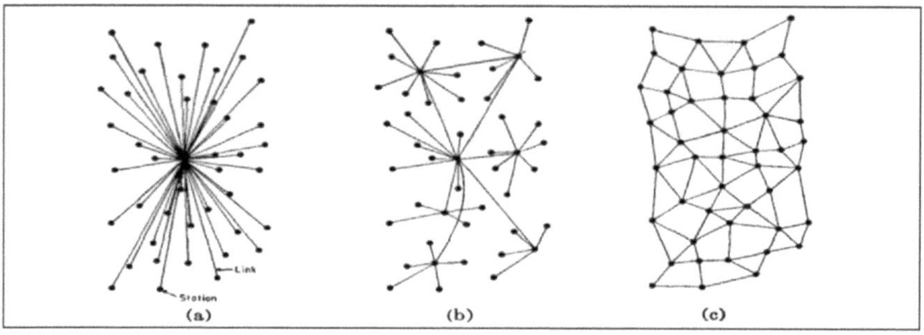

FIGURE 12.3 (a) Centralized; (b) decentralized; and (c) distributed.

12.3.2 TRANSPARENCY

One of the key features of blockchain technology is its visibility. The development of encryption technology allows for greater verification of the technology behind the blockchain, meaning that more users are beginning to trust the network [5].

12.3.2.1 PROVABLY FAIR

One area where blockchain technology really shows its transparency is the Bitcoin casino website. In any casino, the house will still have good, potentially relevant games, allowing users to check the main game server to ensure that the results obtained are real and relevant. This is a real turning point for online gaming, and it is something that casino websites and gaming platforms hope to unite to build a new level of trust between the site and its users to play.

12.3.2.2 PRIVACY

Privacy is one of the most common questions people have when it comes to open blockchain. How can technology demonstrate that blockchain users are anonymous? Interestingly, since not all behaviors can be obtained anonymously, consumers are more willing to communicate with technology, and its anonymity allows the blockchain to maintain transparency. Although all online transactions can be tracked and maintained, the privacy of technology is an important reason for its increasing importance. And help to ensure the reliability of the technology.

12.3.2.3 FULLY AUDITED AND ASSESSMENT RESULTS

While the technology has a high degree of independence, the communication module provides unprecedented transparency in terms of audit completion and practicality. All transactions on this site are indelible, which means that data saved after any network authentication cannot be tampered with, modified, or deleted. If transactions on the network are altered, all other blocks in the system must also be changed, making the entire transaction process impossible. Automatic verification is a key component of the blockchain network, and this eliminates the need for manual verification and measurement.

12.3.2.4 NO ORGANIZATION CONTROL

Because a business is connected to a blockchain network, no organization can control or regulate the network in any way. Blockchain technology is developed around peers, which means that ordinary users from all over the world, known as "miners," have a responsibility to ensure, look for any changes. This allows the platform to be transparent and extremely reliable, allowing many users to make great strides in integrating blockchain technology as part of their daily lives.

12.3.3 IMMUTABILITY

The variance is always defined because the power of the blockchain ledger does not change and therefore the block cannot be changed or switched off. In short, the information in the blockchain cannot be changed [6]. Each block of information (such as fact or detailed information) is generated using cryptographic principles or useful hashes. This value contains a series of numbers made up of individual blocks. Each block has not only the hash or digital signature itself but also the original one. This ensures multiple and uninterrupted merging of blocks. The blockchain technology function ensures that no one can access the system or modify the information stored in the block. It is also important to know that the blocks are distributed and distributed in nature while agreement on the different results contained in the data is reached. This validation agreement of the source information must be saved. There is no doubt that consistency can be a definite plus in this technology. This concept can redefine the entire data review process to be more efficient and cost-effective, and to ensure data integrity and reliability.

12.3.3.1 ACHIEVING IMMUTABILITY

An important component of blockchain is cryptographic hashes. The main advantage of a hash is that it cannot be reversed. That is why it's so popular. The most common hashing function is SHA-256, specifically the

Secure Hash Algorithm 256 where the input is processed into the hash with the output as the final product. In the image below, we can see how the password "Blockchain is distracting" is used as input and then encrypted to produce the output as a checksum [7].

12.3.3.2 ADVANTAGES

The biggest advantage of blockchain is that data cannot be modified, unlike in traditional databases where it is easy to modify and delete data. Furthermore, if any data used is tampered with, the blockchain will be compromised. Making a change results in a broken block and maintaining the status quo poses a significant challenge. When people talk about immutable blockchains, it means that making changes without consensus is difficult, ensuring that information cannot be altered. These techniques have both positive and negative implications for information security. Implementing a new blockchain ledger can guarantee a thorough application process and secure information files. Once the stock market integrates with the blockchain, the data remains there to demonstrate its integrity. Chain integrity can be verified at any time by examining the value of the hash – if there is a discrepancy between block data and hash comparisons, then the alteration is invalid. This enables the organization and its management to detect inaccurate information, ensuring data accuracy.

12.4 FORMS OF BLOCKCHAIN

Blockchain can be classified into two forms: private and public blockchain. Nevertheless, there are also many different types, such as consortium block and hybrid. Each blockchain consists of a constellation of nodes that run on a distributed system. All participants on the network have a copy of the ledger that is immediately updated. Each node can be used to validate, execute, or receive transactions and create blocks [8].

12.4.1 THE PUBLIC BLOCKCHAIN

The public blockchain can be an open, permissionless ledger. Anyone with access to the network can join the blockchain as a validating node.

Participants in the public blockchain can submit new transactions, validate consensus, or perform proof-of-work to add new blocks to the chain. The most common use of public blockchains is for mining and trading cryptocurrencies. Some of the most well-known public blockchains are Bitcoin and Ethereum. Public blockchains are generally secure if users adhere to strict security protocols and procedures. However, there is a risk if participants do not follow security best practices. Examples: Bitcoin, Ethereum, Litecoin.

12.4.2 PRIVATE BLOCKCHAIN

This type of blockchain can be a permissioned or private blockchain that operates within a closed network. Private blockchains are commonly used in organizations or businesses where only authorized members can participate in the network. Security measures, permissions, licenses, and access rights are controlled by the network administrator. Therefore, a private blockchain serves similar purposes as a public one but within a smaller and more controlled environment. Private blockchains are often used for applications like voting, supply chain management, digital identity, asset ownership, and more. Examples of private blockchains include Multichain, Hyperledger (e.g., Sawtooth), Corda, etc.

12.4.3 BLOCKCHAIN ALLIANCE

This form is a semi-distributed type where most organizations manage a blockchain network. Many organizations can serve as a target for this type of blockchain for information exchange or exploration. Blockchain technology is commonly used by banks, government agencies, and others. Examples of integrated blockchains include Web Framework, R3, etc.

12.4.4 HYBRID BLOCKCHAIN

A hybrid blockchain can bridge private and public domains, leveraging the characteristics of both types of blockchains to enable the establishment of a foundational layer without requiring public consensus. Through an interconnected network, users can control access to the data stored in the blockchain. Only specific information or data from the blockchain may be publicly accessible on the website. Hybrid blockchain systems offer great flexibility, allowing users to easily link private blockchains with multiple public blockchains. Transactions within a private blockchain are typically secure within the network. However, users can choose to publish them on the official authentication blockchain. The shared blockchain adds complexity and involves more nodes for verification, enhancing the security and transparency of the network. An example of a hybrid blockchain is Dragonchain.

12.5 IMPORTANCE OF BLOCKCHAIN IN HEALTHCARE

12.5.1 FINANCIAL MANAGEMENT IN HEALTHCARE

Management is not easy, it is not easy to fix, and it is slow. Intermediaries are usually obliged to reconcile the development and resolve arguments. Generally, this involves much cost and effort. Contrasted to conventional techniques, users find the block stingier, clearer, and much more effective. More and more financial facilities are employing this scheme to bring novelties, like intelligent bonds. All healthcare organizations have been engrossed with the blockchain for quite some time now beyond their million-dollar investment and pilot projects. Business procedures are always costly and perilous. In this development, any external entity, like a dealer or agent, collects information, leaving room to make a mistake. Blockchain reduces errors in hiding your books. At the same time, it simplifies the process and eliminates the need for a mediator [9].

12.5.2 HEALTHCARE

Blockchain plays an important role in healthcare because personal health information is stored on the blockchain securely. Only authorized individuals can access this information. This approach can help ensure safer and more effective research while complying with HIPAA regulations. Additionally, medical invoices can be stored on the blockchain and automatically sent to insurance companies for verification. Blockchain technology can also be utilized for general health management, including drug management, control systems, testing, and medical equipment management.

12.5.3 PAYMENT AND TRANSACTIONS

One of the most popular uses of blockchain technology is the fast transfer of funds between parties, making money transfers quicker. By eliminating banks from the process and enabling 24/7 exchanges, most mobile blockchain transactions can be completed within minutes. International payments, which are often error-prone, expensive, and involve borrowing money, can take up to five working days to process. With blockchain technology, real-time transactions can be easily completed without the need for banks, potentially reducing transaction fees [10, 11].

12.5.4 GOVERNMENT

Computer-savvy individuals suggest that protesters could attack electronic devices to manipulate voting. Since the vote is encrypted, the leader is limited. All voters can easily verify if their vote is counted and can still determine who they voted for. This approach also saves money for the government. Blockchain establishes a solid foundation for highly sensitive accessible data. Beginners will be able to use this knowledge to detect fraudulent schemes, and farmers will be able to implement appropriate farming methods. This information is made available to the public throughout the year. Blockchain can share this information with the public at any time. Additionally, it offers the government independent oversight of organizations, NGOs, and institutions.

12.5.5 DATA STANDARDIZATION AND SCOPE

It is crucial for an organization to determine which data will be stored on the Blockchain. In healthcare, the amount of data to be stored on the blockchain is important. The performance of blockchain will be affected by unnecessary transactions if all doctors' notes are stored on the blockchain. Storing demographic data, medical care logs, etc., could enhance operational efficiency. Organizations require a blockchain storage framework to manage performance and standardize data storage by considering the size and format of data. Data size can be managed using technical APIs and implementing big data mechanisms.

12.5.6 MONITOR SUPPLY CHAINS

Providing an optional blockchain can be helpful, especially when it comes to inspecting chains. Now companies can fix shortages in their deliveries quickly and inspect goods in real time. The blockchain will authenticate the companies and consumers to understand how they are producing commodities from well-managed ideas that they believe are made from the very beginning for the consumer. Consumers can use the blockchain to find the source of what they want to buy. In this case, they will also receive assistance from the development block. These companies make it easy for companies to verify the legitimacy of their products using blockchain techniques. For example, it permits corporations to check from the supply chain to the end by providing information about the supply chain and the state when it is transported to the free world. According to the Forbes report, the food industry employs blockchain to trace routes and ensure food safety in its end-user areas.

12.5.7 CRYPTOCURRENCY

Blockchain technology creates a cryptocurrency perspective in the form of Bitcoin. Currency, like the US dollar, is legalized and regulated by the government, usually run by a bank or agency. If something goes wrong, the consumer's bank may fail or they reside in a country with an unstable government, then the consumer's value will deteriorate. These concerns gave birth to bitcoin. Now Blockchain has done its job of allowing bitcoin and other cryptocurrencies to operate without central control by expanding computer network operations. This, of course, reduces the amount of risk, but also eliminates costs and exchange rates. This provides countries with flexible and cost-effective solutions.

12.5.8 SMART CONTRACTS

In the smart contract, the smart contract is embedded in the technical module for contract verification. It works in accordance with specific restrictions that users must agree to. When the terms of the contract are contacted, the stipulations of the contract are ensured to be met. Blockchain meets the obligations of external entities, also safeguarding all ledger participants know the aspects of the contract. The stipulations of the contract are implemented spontaneously when the terms are expired. One can utilize smart contracts designed for various activities, such as financing, basic insurance, property rights, and making financial contracts.

12.5.9 DIGITAL ID

According to the World Bank, there exist more than 1.1 billion people in the world whose identities cannot be identified. At the same time, financial bodies are compelled to abide by the scheme of KYC to obtain detailed information about their customers. Many suppliers have yet to meet these standards properly. To make matters worse, rules vary between borders and regions. Many large companies like Microsoft and Cisco have used blockchain technology to guarantee safety and protection for their customers.

12.5.10 BLOCKCHAIN AND IOT

According to Gartner, about 26 billion IoT devices will be in operation by the end of 2026. The IoT market is expected to grow to $3 trillion every year. Blockchain-enabled smart devices will be faster and more reliable, providing a low level of financial management systems, Internet access, and licensing for users and businesses. Helium utilizes the power of web technologies to connect everything on the internet through blockchain, wireless, and open-source software [12, 13].

12.6 BLOCKCHAIN SECURITY FOR HEALTHCARE

Blockchain technology creates a data structure with computational security advantages. Based on the principles of confidentiality, decentralization, and consensus, it ensures trust in transactions. In most blockchain or distributed ledger technology, data is divided into blocks, with each block containing a record or distribution of objects on the network. Each new block links all the previous blocks in an encrypted chain in an almost immutable manner. All blocks are verified and validated through a consensus mechanism to ensure the authenticity and integrity of each transaction [13, 14]. Blockchain technology enables power distribution among participants in a decentralized network, eliminating single points of failure and preventing clients from altering transaction data.

12.6.1 DEVELOPING ENTERPRISE BLOCKCHAIN SECURITY

When building a blockchain, it is important to consider security in every aspect of blockchain technology, as well as how to manage governance and website. The enterprise's comprehensive blockchain security strategy includes the use of traditional security management and technical management. Other safeguards for a blockchain business solution include:

- Individuality and contact management;
- Strategic management;
- Data privacy;
- Reliable and authenticated communication;
- Intelligent treaty protection;
- Transaction commendation.

12.6.2 BLOCKCHAIN SECURITY GUIDELINES AND BEST PRACTICES

Planning a blockchain solution may need to consider these questions:

- What is the governance model for participating organizations or members?
- What will data be captured in each block?
- What are the relevant regulatory requirements, and how can they be met?
- How are the details of identity managed? Are block payloads encrypted? How are the keys managed and revoked?
- What is the disaster recovery plan for the blockchain participants?
- What is the minimal security posture for blockchain clients for participation?
- What is the logic for resolving blockchain block collisions?

As soon as you start building a blockchain, ensure the safety and security of the location chosen. Choosing low-tech technologies for business needs and operations can stabilize data because of the six gaps. Consider business risk and management. Business risk includes financial, reputational, and business risk. Management risks often stem from blockchain distribution, requiring full management decision-making standards, management guidelines, route identification, and access. Blockchain Security refers to understanding and managing risk on the blockchain network. The decision to implement security in that control builds a blockchain defense standard [15]. Establish a blockchain defense standard to certify every step is taken to have enough blockchain solutions. To realize a blockchain defense standard, managers need to build a risk template that contemplates all business, regulatory, expertise, and practice risks. Later, they ought to weigh the danger to the blockchain and make a threat paradigm. The supervisor requires outlining safety measures to diminish risks and threats created in the resulting areas:

- Implementation of block-specific protection;
- Use of standard security;
- Use business management for blockchain.

12.7 SCOPE AND CHALLENGES OF RESEARCH

12.7.1 BLOCKCHAIN COMPLEXITY

The magnificence of the blockchain rests in the convolution of the network. The more people involved in the business, the better the usability of the blockchain. In the beginning, many PoCs did not survive and ran with little labor cost and expense, as only a few of them had access to the blockchain. Moreover, most companies and banks are now adopting blockchain in their shares. These institutions did not adopt a centralized or integrated approach but adopted a collaborative approach. It increases efficiency due to great efficiency. Many companies need to employ fanatical blockchain consultants, irrespective of whether their active applications are trivial. Second, a specific blockchain function cannot be effortlessly imitated between implementation and credit usage. Each application entails a graver insight of business constraints, and for functions such as insurance agreements and nationwide registers, blockchain can be very diverse [16].

12.7.2 ASTRONOMICAL ENERGY UTILIZATION

Bitcoins are well-known blockchain products. Bitcoin Core should provide almost 200 GB of storage for each blockchain network base. Other requirements include a 5 GB download and a daily 500 MB download.

As India continues to struggle to roll out Bharatmala Broadband and 4 G projects with capacity and power across the country, the use of the blockchain will certainly require improved infrastructure. As far as the Bitcoin blockchain is concerned, energy consumption is still the most important factor for mining workers. Researchers from the University of Cambridge speculated that Bitcoin consumes more energy resources than Switzerland. Strong ideas empower all connections in life. Blockchain only, if we use more communication, please consider this question.

12.7.3 *SCALABILITY CHALLENGES*

Scalability can be termed as another issue and challenge in addition to several applications of blockchains. For example, let us compare the larger central Visa payment system and the larger cryptographic Bitcoin. If Visa can cope with 65,000 transactions per second, the maximum value of Bitcoin is 7 transactions per second. In the case of a centralized architecture, the process is defined by the focal body, not unnecessarily informing other partners of the transaction. This saves time and speed. As for blockchain, make sure to spend a few minutes, as many nodes will allow negotiation. Bitcoin operates on a Proof-of-Work model that is secure but slow at the same time. There is another way to demonstrate share validation, which can ensure quick access but is not a good option for issuing contracts [17].

12.7.4 *BRAIN DRAIN DUE TO BLOCKCHAIN*

Corresponding to various findings and publications, more than 80% of blockchain workers in India are looking for better opportunities. Developers highlighted the appropriate approach because of the country's lack of "constitutional power" in technology blocks. The report shows that blockchain workers have moved to Singapore, the United Arab Emirates, Estonia, and Switzerland, where they are offered tax breaks and incentives to get started. Significant improvements to the digital infrastructure in these countries are more conducive to the use of blockchain. The Indian government recently announced the results of its previous national blockchain blockade, which is likely to be announced soon.

12.8 CONCLUSION

Blockchain technology is revolutionary. It will make life simpler and safer, changing the way personal information is stored and how transactions for goods and services are made. The modern blockchain was made possible with a tremendous number of technological developments through its evolution. Blockchain technology's several models and elements could be largely extensible to a large assortment of circumstances. Several industries and governments have adapted blockchain technology where central control seemed to be inefficient in gaining the trust of users. Soon, we expect to see some innovation in blockchains to improve performance and scalability, which is a special challenge for public blockchains. Along the same lines, there will be new consensus mechanisms going mainstream. For consensus and validation, blockchain researchers are investigating efficient implementation of zero-knowledge proofs and specific variants. Blockchain technology could be quite complementary in a possibility space for the future world that includes both centralized and decentralized models.

KEYWORDS

- **bitcoin**
- **blockchain**
- **cryptocurrency**
- **decentralization**
- **encryption**
- **ledger**
- **privacy**
- **security**
- **transactions**

REFERENCES

1. Sharma, D. K., Kaushik, A. K., Goel, A., & Bhargava, S. (2020). Internet of things and blockchain: Integration, need, challenges, applications, and future scope. In S. Krishnan, V. E. Balas, E. G. Julie, Y. H. Robinson, S. Balaji, & R. Kumar (Eds.),

Handbook of Research on Blockchain Technology (pp. 271–294). Academic Press. https://doi.org/10.1016/B978-0-12-819816-2.00011-3.
2. Sharma, M., Pant, S., Sharma, D. K., Gupta, K. D., Vashishth, V., & Chhabra, A. (2020). Enabling security for the industrial Internet of Things using deep learning, blockchain, and coalitions. *Transactions on Emerging Telecommunications Technologies*, *32*(7), e4137. https://doi.org/10.1002/ett.4137.
3. Khan, P. W., & Byun, Y. (2020). A blockchain-based secure image encryption scheme for the industrial Internet of Things. *Entropy, 22*(2), 175. https://doi.org/10.3390/e22020175.
4. Zarrin, J., Wen Phang, H., Babu Saheer, L., & Zarrin, B., (2021). Blockchain for decentralization of internet: prospects, trends, and challenges. *Cluster Computing, 24*(4), 2841–2866.
5. Centobelli, P., Cerchione, R., Del Vecchio, P., Oropallo, E., & Secundo, G., (2022). Blockchain technology for bridging trust, traceability and transparency in circular supply chain. *Information & Management, 59*(7), p.103508.
6. Kaushiki Srivastav, (2019). "A Guide to Blockchain Immutability and Challenges," Dzone.com, 29 March, https://dzone.com/articles/a-guide-to-blockchain-immutability-and-chief-chall.
7. Rahardja, U., Hidayanto, A. N., Lutfiani, N., Febiani, D. A. & Aini, Q., (2021). Immutability of Distributed Hash Model on Blockchain Node Storage. *Sci. J. Informatics, 8*(1), 137–143.
8. Wei, Q., Li, B., Chang, W., Jia, Z., Shen, Z. and Shao, Z., (2022). A survey of blockchain data management systems. *ACM Transactions on Embedded Computing Systems (TECS), 21*(3), 1–28.
9. Cuel, R., & Gabriella, C., (2019). In vino veritas? Wine industry and Blockchain. In Proceedings of ITAIS and MCIS 2019: a joint event: the 13th Mediterranean Conference on Information Systems and the 16th Conference of the Italian Chapter of AIS. ITHUM and ITAIS.
10. Sharma, D. K., Pant, S., Sharma, M., & Brahmachari, S. (2020). Cryptocurrency mechanisms for blockchains: Models, characteristics, challenges, and applications. In S. Krishnan, V. E. Balas, E. G. Julie, Y. H. Robinson, S. Balaji, & R. Kumar (Eds.), *Handbook of research on blockchain technology* (pp. 323–348). Academic Press. https://doi.org/10.1016/B978-0-12-819816-2.00013-7.
11. Sharma, D. K., Pardhe, T., Kulshreshtha, Y., & Singh, S. (2020). Blockchain applications and implementation. In *Handbook of IoT and Blockchain* (pp. 95–118). CRC Press.
12. Dulhare, U. N., & Rasool, S. (2019). IoT evolution and security challenges in cyber space: IoT security. In S. Geetha & A. V. Phamila (Eds.), *Countering Cyber Attacks and Preserving the Integrity and Availability of Critical Systems* (pp. 99–127). IGI Global.
13. Riyal, A., Prasad, P. S., & Sharma, D. K. (2021). Internet of things and blockchain amalgamation, requirements, issues, and practices. In *Blockchain Technology for Data Privacy Management* (p. 23). CRC Press.
14. Alshehri, M., (2023). Blockchain-assisted cyber security in medical things using artificial intelligence. *Electron. Res. Arch, 31*(2), 708–728.

15. Rasool, S., & Dulhare, U. N. (2022). Data center security. In *Green Computing in Network Security: Energy Efficient Solutions for Business and Home* (1st edn.). CRC Press. https://doi.org/10.1201/9781003097198.
16. Banyal, S., Saxena, M., & Sharma, D. K. (2020). Blockchain-enabled security and privacy schemes in IoT technologies. In *Handbook of IoT and Blockchain* (p. 24). CRC Press.
17. Dulhare, U. N., & Rasool, S. (2022). Smart airport system to counter COVID-19 and future sustainability. In C. Satyanarayana, X. Z. Gao, C. Y. Ting, & N. B. Muppalaneni (Eds.), *Machine Learning and Internet of Things for Societal Issues: Advanced Technologies and Societal Change* (pp. 5–20). Springer. https://doi.org/10.1007/978-981-16-5090-1_5.

Index

B

E

G

H

I

M

S

T

U

V

W

X

Y

Z